An academic contribution
from the
Ludwig J. Pyrtek Chair
in surgery

# SURGICAL BLUNDERS

## AND HOW TO AVOID THEM

# SURGICAL BLUNDERS

## AND HOW TO AVOID THEM

By Frumius Bandersnatch, M.D.

TRIAD PUBLISHING COMPANY
GAINESVILLE, FLORIDA

Printed in the United States of America

*Library of Congress Cataloging-in-Publication Data*

Bandersnatch, Frumius.
Surgical blunders and how to avoid them / by Frumius Bandersnatch.
p. cm.
ISBN 0-937404-31-4
1. Surgical errors--Anecdotes. 2. Surgical errors--Prevention.
I. Title.
RD27.85.B36 1990 89-5082
617--dc20 CIP

*Published and distribtuted by Triad Publishing Co., Inc., 1110 NW Eighth Ave. Gainesville, FL 32601. For information on bulk orders write Special Sales Dept.*

Illustrations by Louis

# CONTENTS

# PREFACE

THIS BOOK IS A COLLECTION of anecdotes about mistakes that have been made by surgeons. Some of these are humorous, some are embarrassing, and others are tragic. All of the stories are true, but in many the details were changed to prevent the perpetrator from being too easily identified.

Every surgeon, except of course the author, has made mistakes from time to time. Most of the errors related in this book could have been prevented if their possibility had been recognized prospectively. The surgeons who committed them have filed them under "stupid mistakes I have made that I will never make again," and indeed, this type of error is rarely repeated in the same form by the same individual. However, sooner or later someone else will repeat the mistake unless he has had the opportunity to experience the error vicariously either by watching it happen or by reading this book. It has been said that good judgment comes from experience and that experience comes from bad judgment.

The author has had extensive experience in nearly all fields of surgery. Although he, himself, has never made a mistake, he has observed many mistakes that have been made by others. Some of these anecdotes were collected from friends of the author who have also never made any mistakes but have knowledge of mistakes made by others. Although it is customary to acknowledge contributors to medical books, in this case they all declined the honor.

One of the rituals of surgical practice is the complications conference. It is a traditional practice at these conferences to classify errors into categories of diagnosis, judgment, technique, or management. I have used these categories and added two of my own to organize this book. Some of the cases could fit in more than one category, and the classification is often arbitrary.

It is also a tradition of these conferences to assign blame, usually to the lowest ranking member of the housestaff who could be stuck with it. In some places the residents are expected to stop by the carpenter's shop before the conference to be measured for a cross. When I was a resident, I took a 44 oak. In this book I have tried to avoid this practice and let the darts hit where they will. He who is without stones may cast the first sin.

F. B.

# ONE

# ERRORS IN TECHNIQUE

ERRORS IN TECHNIQUE are problems in execution. The surgeon may have made a correct diagnosis and may have exercised good judgment in matching the patient to the correct operation; however, in carrying out that procedure, something goes wrong.

None of the "ETs" reported in this section was due to a lack of skill, but rather to a momentary lapse in attention to detail. An operation is more than the sum of its parts, but each part still has the potential to ruin the entire result.

It is often the routine steps in operations that are most vulnerable to error. Some of these steps are so routine that they are practiced almost without thought, and the surgeon may let his guard down and start thinking about his next fishing trip.

Some errors in technique come from trying to take shortcuts (no pun intended).

Some errors in technique are the result of earlier errors in diagnosis or judgment.

But whatever the cause, they are out there waiting for

you. Just when you thought it was safe to go back in the operating room . . . . Zap!

Errors in technique will continue as long as operations are done by human surgeons, and maybe even after they are someday done by robots. When you read these and are tempted to chuckle at the dummys who made them, remember that there but for the grace of God . . . .

## *1. The Importance of Adequate Exposure*

The patient was a severely debilitated elderly man with an unresectable cancer of the esophagus. Because he was unable to take any nourishment by mouth and a feeding tube was deemed impractical, it was elected to place a gastrostomy. Because of his severely debilitated condition, a small incision and a local anesthetic were used.

The day after the procedure was performed, the patient promptly developed bowel sounds and, therefore, it was elected to start his tube feeding. Immediately after the tube feeding was begun, the nurse called the physician to report that the patient was having excessive watery diarrhea. This was initially attributed to the hyperosmolar tube feeding formula, and therefore the feedings were diluted and the rate was decreased.

However, diarrhea continued to be a problem. On subsequent abdominal X-rays, it was repeatedly noticed that there was no gas bubble in the stomach, but there was considerable gas and distention of the colon. This led to a contrast study of the "gastrostomy," which showed the gastrostomy tube was, in fact, in the transverse colon.

This error was clearly one of trying to minimize an operation by using the smallest possible incision, and this led to inadequate surgical exposure.

The first three rules of surgery are:

1. Exposure.
2. Exposure.
3. Exposure.

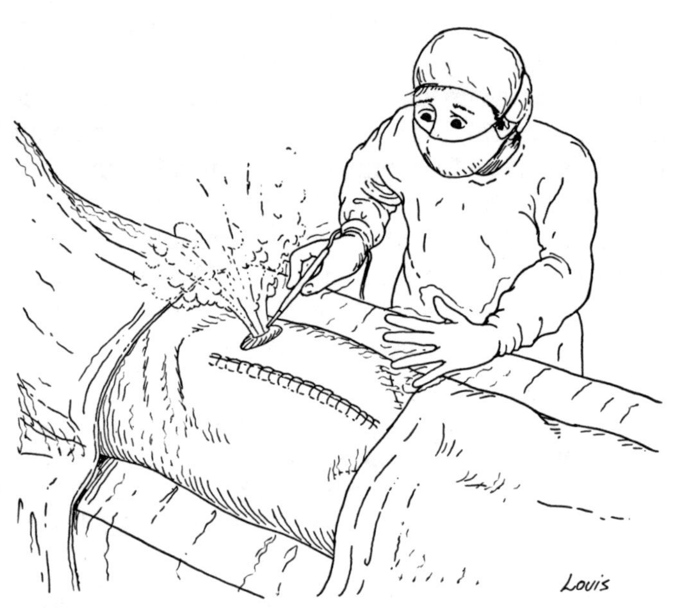
Louis

## 2. *The Case of the Embarrassing Explosion*

The patient was an elderly man with an advanced carcinoma of the rectum. It had been determined that the tumor was too advanced to be resectable, so the plan was to treat it with radiation therapy and manage his symptoms of bowel obstruction with a loop colostomy.

The bowel was prepared as well as possible under the circumstances. The transverse colon was exposed through a midline incision and a transverse loop colostomy was brought out through a small muscle-splitting incision in the left upper quadrant. The midline wound was then closed and it was elected to open the transverse colon loop to provide the earliest possible relief of the patient's distention.

The loop was incised longitudinally using a Bovie. Immediately upon entering the lumen, there was a loud explosion, which was evidently produced by ignition of bowel gas. Fortunately, the only serious damage was done to the surgeon's ego and wearing apparel.

## 3. *The Upside Down Kidney*

A 29-year-old chronic renal failure patient was undergoing renal transplantation with a related living donor. The vascular portion of the procedure went quite well and the kidney appeared to be perfusing well; but when the ureteroneocystostomy was done, the ureter seemed to kink at the ureteral pelvic junction.

On closer inspection, it became apparent the kidney was in upside down, causing the ureter to come off at an inappropriate angle. This was a significant problem and required takedown of both vascular repairs, which were subsequently redone.

There were no other problems and the patient did well.

## 4. *The Tube Hepatostomy*

A 32-year-old man was brought to the emergency room after an automobile accident in which he sustained blunt trauma to the chest. The chest X-ray showed multiple rib fractures on the right side and a hemopneumothorax. The patient's vital signs were stable, and a closed tube thoracostomy was planned.

A small incision was made on the right side in the midaxillary line at about what was thought to be the level of the seventh rib. When the chest tube was introduced bluntly, the suction failed to produce much bloody drainage, and followup X-rays showed the chest still contained a large amount of blood. A second chest tube was placed a little higher and this tube evacuated the hemothorax and expanded the lung.

By now, the patient was developing some signs of abdominal tenderness, primarily in the right upper quadrant. Therefore, an abdominal tap was done, which demonstrated bleeding within the abdominal cavity.

At laparotomy, it was found that the chest tube was entering the right side of the liver. There were no other intra-abdominal injuries. It was apparent that the first chest tube had been placed too low and had passed through the diaphragm and entered the liver. Fortunately, withdrawal of the tube was all that was necessary, and the patient made an uneventful recovery.

The lesson to be learned from this case is that it is very dangerous to place a chest tube low in the chest. A similar injury, which has been known to occur when a chest tube is placed on the left side, is rupture of the spleen. In general, it is probably best to place the tube no lower than the sixth intercostal space and, perhaps, to lower the diaphragm by having the patient take a deep breath as the tube enters the chest. It is also probably a good idea to direct the tube in a cephalad direction; this is unnecessary if the pleural space is opened to direct vision so that the surgeon can see that the diaphragm is not being penetrated.

## *5. Safe Surgery Requires Adequate Anesthesia*

A 16-year-old girl had undergone successful renal transplantation, and it was decided to remove her external hemodialysis shunt. The shunt had been placed from the posterior tibial artery just above the medial malleolus to the adjacent saphenous vein.

The patient was taken to the minor surgery suite, where, under local anesthesia, the previous incision over the posterior tibial artery was opened and the posterior tibial artery was exposed. In spite of repeated injections of the anesthetic, the patient remained agitated, and she complained of a great deal of pain in the operative site. A considerable amount of capillary bleeding obscured the operative field.

After a prolonged and difficult struggle, the catheter was removed. There was brisk arterial bleeding from the puncture site. A right angle clamp was passed around the posterior tibial artery and the vessel was ligated with 3-0 silk. The wound was closed and the patient was returned to the ward, where she promptly reported that the bottom of her foot — the entire sole and the plantar surface of the toes — was numb.

Therefore, the following day the patient was returned to the operating room, where, with a general anesthetic and a proximal tourniquet, the wound was explored. It was found that the proximal ligature had encircled not only the posterior tibial artery but also the posterior tibial nerve. This ligature was removed and a new, more selective ligature was applied to the posterior tibial artery.

An analysis of this apparently technical error showed that it probably occurred because the magnitude of the procedure was underestimated. The patient was an anxious individual and was therefore a questionable candidate for local anesthesia. Local anesthetics are also somewhat difficult to use in previously operated sites because of their poor diffusion through scar tissue.

A general or regional anesthetic would have allowed the use of a proximal tourniquet, which would have made visibility and accurate surgical exposure more feasible. Viewed in retrospect, a general anesthetic and the use of a tourniquet might seem excessive for this apparently minor procedure, but would have prevented a significant complication.

## *6. A Difficult Problem in the Extubation*

The patient was a 26-year-old man who had been involved in a major automobile accident and was brought to the emergency room with problems related to multiple trauma. He had a skull fracture, several contusions, multiple facial fractures, multiple rib fractures, an unstable chest, and fractures of both legs.

After resuscitation and stabilization, the patient was taken to the operating room where he was simultaneously managed by four different surgical services. One team operated on the skull fractures, another on the facial fractures, and a third on the lower extremity fractures. Anesthesia was administered through a nasotracheal tube. In addition to appropriate management of his skull fractures, a depressed zygomatic maxillary fracture on one side had to be reduced and stablized; this was done using a Kirschner wire, which was passed from one side of the face to the other.

Because of the patient's unstable chest wall, the nasotracheal tube was left in place when he was taken to the intensive care unit, where he was kept on a ventilator until his respiratory status stabilized. It was then decided to remove the nasotracheal tube; however, the resident found he was unable to remove it. A more thorough examination of the nasotracheal tube showed that the Kirschner wire used to stabilize the facial fractures had passed through the tube on its way across the face. Removal of the Kirschner wire greatly facilitated removal of the nasotracheal tube.

Fortunately, the fracture proved to have adequate stablity without the wire and, therefore, there were no major consequences to this error.

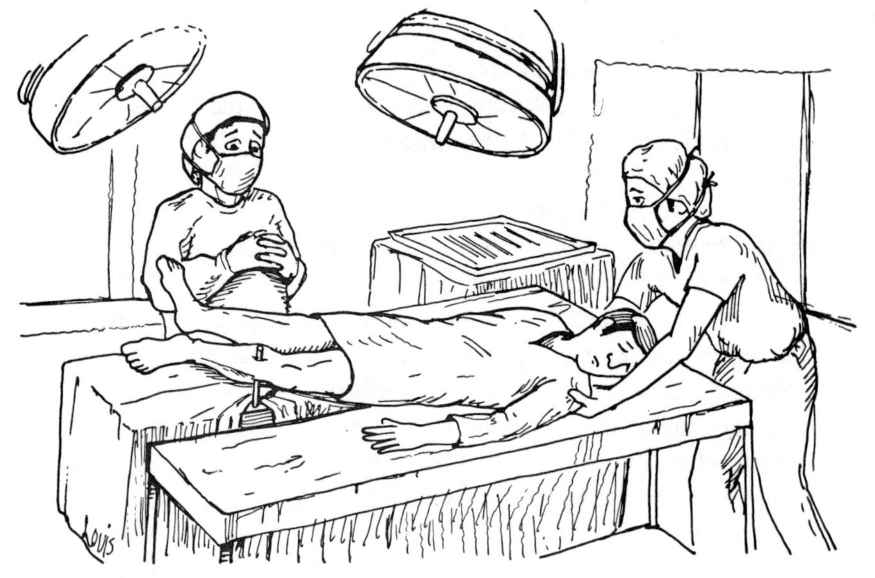
Louis

## 7. *Nailing Down the Problem*

A 29-year-old man was involved in a motorcycle accident and was brought to the emergency room with an open fracture of the femur and other major injuries, including a ruptured spleen.

The patient was under anesthesia for exploratory laparotomy. There was not enough room for the orthopedic surgeon to work comfortably at the same time, but it was late at night and he did not want to wait until the general surgeons were finished.

The orthopedist elected to manage the fracture initially with skeletal traction, and after the wounds had been adequately debrided and closed, he placed a Steinmann pin through the proximal tibia by using a power drill, and because of the crowded conditions he had to reach under the drapes to use the drill.

Long after the orthopedist had gone, when it was time to remove the patient from the table, it was found that he was firmly attached to the table by the pin that had been drilled not only through the bone, but well into the table.

The problem was easily solved with a pin cutter, and resulted in no significant difficulty thereafter.

## 8. *The Blunt Esophagectomy*

A 45-year-old man was admitted to the hospital with a long history of heartburn and a recent onset of dysphagia. Prior to admission he had had an upper gastrointestinal series that demonstrated gastroesophageal reflux and distal ulcerations in the esophagus, with mucosal changes indicative of Barrett's esophagus. These findings were confirmed on esophagoscopy, and the plan was to correct the patient's gastroesophageal reflux.

At operation, the surgeon was mobilizing the stomach and the distal esophagus through the somewhat enlarged esophageal hiatus. There was a significant inflammation in the area of the gastroesophageal junction, and visibility was limited by some bleeding in the area.

The surgeon elected to sweep his finger around the esophagus by blunt dissection and, as he did that, he pulled distally on the stomach, only to feel it suddenly give and to discover that he was holding the bloody stump of a stomach in his hand. The end of the esophagus was, meanwhile, retracting into the posterior mediastinum. Obviously, what happened was that the stomach had been avulsed from the distal esophagus, making the surgical treatment of this patient substantially more complex.

The lesson in this story is that patients with severe distal esophagitis and ulceration usually have a very friable esophagus that can be easily torn. The usual amount of trauma and tugging that is endured by the esophagus during mobilization for vagotomy will not be tolerated by an esophagus that has enough reflux esophagitis to develop Barrett's esophagus.

## *9. The Case of the Choledochol-Caval Shunt*

The patient was a 47-year-old alcoholic with moderately severe Laennec's cirrhosis. He had been admitted to the medical service with upper gastrointestinal bleeding.

At endoscopy, he was found to have bleeding from the esophageal varices. These were initially controlled with a balloon tube. The bleeding recurred, however, so surgical consultation was requested for treatment of his portal hypertension.

At surgery, the vena cava was exposed with difficulty because of bleeding from large retroperitoneal veins. The surgeon recalled afterward that the field was obscured with a great deal of blood and that he had had difficulty getting his assistants to retract adequately for good exposure. The "portal vein" was then exposed, but when it was opened there was no blood within the lumen. Since the vein had been clamped proximally and distally, very little concern was noted at the time. A standard side-to-side anastomosis was done. The post-shunt portal vein pressure was not measured, but the mesenteric veins were observed to remain distended.

The day following the operation, the patient had recurrent bleeding and was noted to have substantially increased jaundice. However, on endoscopy the bleeding did not appear to be coming from the esophageal varices, and no ulcers were noted in the stomach. It was therefore decided to re-explore the patient for the possibility that an ulceration somewhere was causing the bleeding.

On re-exploration it was found that the anastomosis had actually been made between the vena cava and the common bile duct, and this was causing bleeding through the bile duct into the duodenum. It was also noted that the choledochol-caval shunt had not resulted in any significant improvement in the portal hypertension. A takedown of this anastomosis and an anastomosis of the vena cava to the portal vein resulted in considerable improvement of the patient's condition.

This case once again illustrates the importance of good exposure and identification of anatomy. Just knowing that this complication is possible should be enough to prevent its recurrence.

## *10. The Case of the Loop Gastrostomy*

The patient was a 63-year-old man with a long history of diverticulitis. He had not done well on medical management. On the day prior to admission he had had progressive onset of severe left lower quadrant pain, nausea, vomiting, and high fever.

At the initial examination he had a tender mass in the left lower quadrant, his temperature was 38.5 degrees orally, and his white count was 23,000. An upright X-ray of the abdomen showed some extralumenal gas in the left lower quadrant with air fluid levels. A tentative diagnosis of a perforated sigmoid diverticulum with abscess was made, and it was elected to manage this with a small left lower quadrant incision for drainage of the abscess.

Prior to the incision and drainage, a separate incision was made in the left upper quadrant for a loop colostomy. The left upper quadrant incision was about three inches long, and the surgeon noticed that he had a little more difficulty than usual in bringing the colon loop into the wound. The colostomy was opened at the time of operation and a colostomy bag was placed over it.

During the following 48 hours it was noted that the patient failed to have adequate improvement and continued to have fever and feculent drainage from the left lower quadrant. It was also noted that his colostomy had not had any output except for a small amount of clear fluid.

On the third postoperative day, while irrigating the nasogastric tube, it was found that fluid was being expelled into the colostomy bag. At this point a problem was suspected and later confirmed. As you have probably already guessed, the patient had not, in fact, undergone a loop colostomy but had undergone a loop gastrostomy.

This again illustrates the importance of adequate exposure for a surgical procedure. Because of the small size of the incision, the surgeon had mistaken the stomach for the transverse colon.

## *11. The Case of the Median Nerve Tendon Graft*

A 32-year-old sheet metal worker had injured his right fifth finger when a sharp piece of sheet metal fell on it, lacerating the flexor tendons and fracturing the proximal phalanx. Because of the unfavorable nature of the tendon laceration, it was decided to repair only the fracture at the time of the initial injury. This was done by open reduction and internal fixation.

After the fracture healed and the patient regained some of his passive flexion, a flexor tendon graft was done using the palmaris longus tendon. The surgeon noted the tendon graft had an unusually soft texture. Following the procedure, the patient complained of numbness in his hand.

The patient was referred to another surgeon who, on his examination, found signs of a complete median nerve paralysis at the level of the distal forearm. On exploration, the second surgeon found that the median nerve had been removed for a distance of about 15 cm, and this required reconstruction with nerve grafts. In addition, the finger was completely stiff. On exploration of the finger, he found that there were remnants of the median nerve present in the tendon sheath. The final functional result was very poor, as might be expected.

In retrospect, it is quite obvious that the first surgeon mistook the median nerve for the palmaris longus tendon and removed it as a tendon graft. Not only does the median nerve make a very poor substitute for tendon, its removal has other very serious adverse effects on hand function.

Obviously, the error was in obtaining the graft through a small incision and using a tendon stripper without adequately defining the anatomy. The patient was one of the 15 percent of the normal population that has no palmaris longus tendon. This should have been easily determined on pre-operative exam.

## *12. An Unorthodox Retroperitoneal Drain*

At approximately 2:00 A.M. the intern was called to see a patient who had pulled out his nasogastric tube. The patient was an elderly man who was agitated and confused. The intern had a great deal of difficulty passing the tube, and he later related that it had taken several attempts and somewhat more force than usual.

The following morning it was noticed on rounds that there had not been any gastric juice returned from the tube, and the patient appeared to have a distended stomach. Several attempts to irrigate and reposition the tube did not succeed in correcting the problem. Some air was injected into the tube, but auscultation over the abdomen during the injection of air did not give the characteristic bubbling sound that would be expected when the tube is properly placed.

An X-ray of the abdomen was obtained. On casual inspection of this X-ray, the tube appeared to be in the correct location just below the diaphragm. However, on more careful inspection of the X-ray it was noticed that there was air contrast around the psoas muscles.

The patient was re-examined and it was noticed that the tube had punctured the posterior pharynx and then evidently had passed through the retropharyngeal space, through the posterior mediastinum, and into the retroperitoneum. The tube was removed and, fortunately, there were no significant consequences from this misadventure.

There are several lessons to be learned from this case, not the least of which is that a relatively stiff plastic tube can do more damage than one might anticipate. Another important point to remember is that passing a nasogastric tube in an uncooperative patient has a significant potential for disaster.

## *13. The Case of the Iatrogenic Stab Wound to the Abdomen*

A 24-year-old man was brought to the emergency room after a motorcycle accident. He had an obvious fracture of the femur and left upper quadrant abdominal pain. His hematocrit was 36 percent and his vital signs were stable.

On examination of the abdomen, there was some moderate tenderness in the left upper quadrant with pain referred to the left shoulder on left upper quadrant palpation. He had a history of a previous stab wound of the abdomen and had undergone exploratory laparotomy shortly after that injury; he had a midline scar from the upper abdomen to just below the umbilicus.

Because of a strong suspicion of a ruptured spleen, it was elected to do a peritoneal lavage to check out the possibility of blood in the peritoneal cavity. A small skin incision was made in the lower abdominal scar just below the umbilicus, and a peritoneal dialysis trocar was used to bluntly enter the peritoneal cavity. Nothing was obtained on aspiration, so 1,000 cc of saline was infused and then drained back into the bottle, demonstrating grossly bloody fluid.

The catheter was removed, and the patient was taken to the operating room, where exploratory laparotomy was done through the old midline scar. He was found to have numerous adhesions of small bowel to the anterior abdominal wall and a large amount of bloody fluid in the abdomen, but examination of the spleen was normal. The bleeding proved to be coming from a small hole in the mesentery, which had obviously been caused by the peritoneal dialysis catheter.

In retrospect, it is obvious that the patient's abdominal

injury was insignificant and the false positive peritoneal lavage was due to a puncture of the small bowel mesentery by the trocar. The most obvious error in this case was in selecting the lower abdominal scar as a puncture site for introduction of the dialysis catheter.

The use of a blunt trocar in a patient who has had a previous laparotomy is a very questionable decision because of the very strong likelihood of adhesions of bowel in general and to the old laparotomy scar in particular. If a peritoneal lavage had been clearly indicated, which it seems to have been, it would have been far more appropriate to use a remote site. In addition, passing the catheter bluntly is significantly more dangerous than making the incision in the peritoneal membrane under direct vision.

In this case the surgeon was indeed fortunate that he had not perforated the bowel itself, causing even more severe complications.

## *14. NG Tube Stapled and Cut*

A 72-year-old man was seen in consultation because of persistent bleeding from a gastric ulcer. All medical efforts to control the bleeding had failed, and therefore it was decided to do a partial gastrectomy.

The distal half of the stomach was removed, using a device that simultaneously staples and cuts the stomach. A gastrojejunostomy was then done using a second stapling device that simultaneously staples and cuts.

The patient initially appeared to be doing reasonably well. On the third post-op day the nasogastric tube was removed with minimal difficulty. However, when it was removed, it was noted that the distal end of it was gone and the cut end of the tube had several staples in it.

Soon afterward, the patient began to develop signs of sepsis, and suture line leak was suspected. Upon re-exploration, the distal end of the nasogastric tube was found loose in the peritoneal cavity and there was a small hole in the gastric stump suture line. This was repaired and the patient went on to recover.

This case illustrates the significant dangers of stapling devices. In any gastrectomy, it is possible to inadvertently cross clamp the nasogastric tube when dividing the stomach. With the older, more conventional suture techniques, the cut tube would obviously be noticed during the suture of the gastric stump.

As clearly demonstrated by this case, a stapling and cutting device is more than capable of transecting a tube without having any noticeable effect on the device. This type of error is very easily prevented simply by withdrawing the tube before transecting the stomach and then palpating the end of the tube, which should be drawn all the way back to the gastroesophageal junction. After the completion of all the anastomoses, the tube can easily be advanced back into the stomach.

## *15. The Roux-en-U*

A 46-year-old woman was referred to a surgeon by a gastroenterologist because of intractable duodenal ulcer.

The surgeon elected to do a vagotomy and partial gastrectomy, and, because of the chronic inflammation around the duodenum, he did not feel that a primary gastroduodenal anastomosis would be safe. Therefore, he elected to re-establish continuity with a gastrojejunostomy, and decided to use a Roux-en-Y.

The patient's early postoperative course was uneventful. However, as soon as she began taking liquids by mouth she immediately had difficulty with vomiting. It was noted that she vomited bile-stained material.

An upper GI X-ray showed no emptying of the stomach. On endoscopy, bile was seen refluxing up through the anastomosis. The endoscopist was able to advance the endoscope easily across the anastomosis, ruling out obstruction.

The surgeon found these symptoms very perplexing, but because of the bile entering the stomach, and on the advice of his consultants, he re-explored the patient. On re-exploration he found that he had inadvertently used the proximal end of the jejunum for anastomosis to the stomach instead of the distal end. A takedown of the anastomic repairs and a rearrangement into the proper sequence corrected the problem.

Analysis of this error shows that it was due to inattention to detail. Once the surgeon had divided the jejunum he became disoriented, but he could easily have avoided this problem had he been thinking about it. Recognizing the error in the post-operative period was difficult; the clues were the presence of bile and the advice of a senior consultant that this error was one that had been known to occur.

## *16. Don't Overestimate the Chief*

The patient was a young man with regional enteritis, who required the resection of two segments of small bowel. The operation left an interpolated segment of about 20 centimeters, which the surgeon elected to preserve in order to maintain as much bowel length as possible in anticipation of future difficulties. Preserving the segment made it necessary to do two intestinal anastomoses.

The procedure was somewhat unusual in that it was performed by the chief of the department, assisted only by a medical student; all the housestaff were occupied elsewhere. As the anastomoses were being done, the student observed that the segment of bowel was rotated 180 degrees, which would reverse peristalsis. Although he was somewhat puzzled by that, he was intimidated by the unusual situation of being first assistant to the department chairman, so he did not question the reason for this unusual step.

As the surgeon began to close the mesentery he noticed his error and had something of a temper outburst, which he directed largely at himself. After a few minutes of swearing he looked up at the student and asked him if he had seen that the bowel was reversed.

The student, not wishing to lie to his chief, answered in the affirmative, and that made the temper tantrum even worse.

The chief then demanded to know why the student did not say something before he had completed both anastomoses.

The student, with more honesty than tact, explained, "Well sir, you're the Chief of Surgery and I just thought you knew what you were doing."

The lesson in this case was for the student; on that day he learned that even the department chairman is capable of making an error.

## *17. Percutaneous Cystostomy for Peritoneal Lavage*

The patient was a 39-year-old man who suffered a severe closed-head injury in an automobile accident. A craniotomy for an epidural hematoma needed to be done, and there was some concern about the possibility of intra-abdominal bleeding because of an otherwise unexplained drop in hematocrit.

After the patient was in the operating room and was turned in the lateral decubitus position for the purpose of having a craniotomy, the neurosurgeon contacted the general surgeon. He had intended to call in the general surgeon earlier but, in his haste to treat the epidural hematoma, had forgotten.

The general surgeon elected to evaluate the abdomen with peritoneal lavage, which was done with what was believed to be a puncture of the peritoneum under direct vision. Clear fluid returned through the cathether, but when the irrigation fluid was run in, the patient was noted to have a substantial increase in urine output, and very little fluid could be recovered from the catheter. A small amount of methylene blue was added to the irrigation fluid, and that also was recovered in the urinary collection bag. The catheter was withdrawn and the patient made an uneventful recovery from the bladder perforation.

In retrospect, it is obvious that the peritoneal lavage catheter was actually a suprapubic cystostomy. The patient had a Foley catheter in place and it was therefore assumed the bladder was decompressed. Obviously this was not the case. A further error in judgment was in performing the peritoneal lavage with the patient on his side. Although this may have contributed to the problem, it could not by itself account for the complication.

Perhaps if a surgeon has occasion to do peritoneal lavage under less than ideal circumstances, he might take an extra moment to make sure the Foley catheter has, in fact, completely emptied the bladder, which this surgeon didn't. Not only that, what he thought was a direct visualization of the peritoneum was obviously a direct visualization of the bladder instead.

## *18. The Case of the Leaning Intern*

The patient was a 59-year-old man with a cancer of the rectum. He was undergoing abdominoperineal resection.

Angled leg holders were mounted to the table and the usual lithotomy position was used. Before the operation the patient was positioned by the chief resident, who fastened a large foam pad around each leg. During the operation everything appeared to be going well. Postoperatively, the patient had an uneventful course until the morning after surgery, when it was discovered that he could not walk. The problem was bilateral foot drop.

It seems the intern had been standing between the patient's legs during the abdominal part of the procedure and was holding retractors from an uncomfortable position. In addition, he had been up most of the preceding night and was very tired. As a result of these factors, he was leaning against the patient's legs during most of the procedure. This appeared to be the cause of the nerve compression injury. Fortunately, the patient recovered within three weeks and had no residual problem.

The lesson to be learned from this case is that the patient is not to be used as a leaning post, and that even foam padding and good positioning prior to surgery do not necessarily protect the patient from peripheral nerve injury.

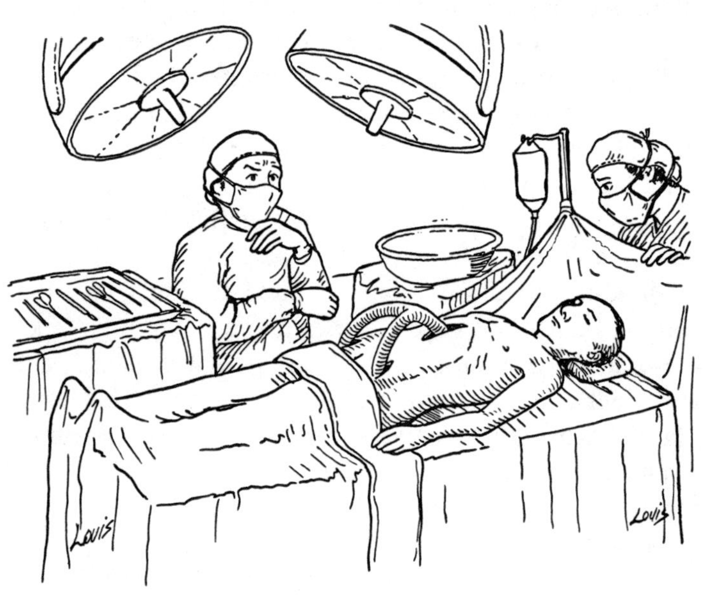
Louis
Louis

## *19. The Case of the Untunneled Bypass Graft*

The patient was a 64-year-old man with severe claudication secondary to distal aortic obstruction. It was elected to bypass the obstruction with a prosthetic graft from the aorta to the common femoral arteries. The procedure went quite well, and as soon as the clamps were removed there was excellent flow through the graft and good distal pulses in both feet.

The only problem was that the graft exited the abdominal wound and then entered each groin wound. The surgeon had forgotten to tunnel the distal limbs of the bifurcation graft. Needless to say, it was necessary to redo the distal anastomoses.

## *20. Adult Tubes Are Not for Babies*

The patient was a newborn male who had undergone emergent cardiac surgery. Postoperatively he developed some gastric distention, so a sump-type nasogastric tube was passed.

The tube failed to decompress the stomach and, in fact, the abdomen became more distended over the next four days. An abdominal film showed the tube curving across the left upper quadrant and the tip of the tube located to the right of the midline. Although the tube was on suction, there was a large air bubble in the stomach.

Because the patient's abdominal signs were getting worse, a pediatric surgeon was asked to see the patient on the fourth postoperative day. He promptly explored the abdomen and found the tube perforating the anterior wall of the antrum and protruding two inches into the peritoneal cavity.

This error was caused by a failure to appreciate the delicacy of the newborn stomach. Sump-type plastic tubes tend to be very stiff, which makes them easier to pass but also makes them more capable of perforating the stomach. A better choice for a small infant is a soft rubber tube.

## *21. The Case of the Upside Down Arch Bar*

The patient was a 23-year-old man who had been involved in a fist fight at a local bar. He had an uncomplicated fracture of the mandible, and it was decided to manage this with arch bars and intermaxillary fixation. The procedure was done under local anesthesia, and it was difficult because the patient was not particularly cooperative.

After both the upper and lower arch bars were in place, it was discovered that both of them were upside down. Because the upper arch bar had lugs pointing down and the lower arch bar had lugs pointing up, the surgeon concluded that he could not apply the fixation wires. He had the patient put under general anesthesia and replaced both arch bars.

Placing the arch bars with the lugs pointing the wrong way is a stupid but understandable mistake. Most surgeons who treat mandible fractures have made this mistake once, although hardly anyone has done it twice. A contributing factor in this case was the inadequate anesthesia.

However, once the mistake had been made, it was not necessary to change the arch bars. Fixation wires could still have been applied by looping the wires over the arch bars.

## *22. The Case of the Migratory Forehead Defect*

The patient was a 25-year-old man who had been in a motorcycle accident and suffered a severe open skull fracture of the right frontal bone involving the superior orbital rim. There was considerable bone loss and some brain injury, but after good debridement and wound care, the patient subsequently made a satisfactory recovery. He was, however, left with a major contour defect of the forehead and orbit.

The surgeon had recently attended a meeting where he had learned of a new technique for bone grafting of the facial skeleton. This new technique involved the use of the outer table of skull as a bone graft rather than the more traditional iliac or rib bone graft.

The patient's wound was re-explored through the original coronal incision, and the defects in the right frontal bone and orbit were thoroughly exposed by subperiosteal dissection. The outer table bone graft was then taken from the left temporal skull, removing only the outer table of bone, which was shaped appropriately and wired in place to correct the orbital and frontal deformity. However, when the skin was redraped it was apparent the patient's receding hairline had resulted in the concavity of the donor site being quite visible on the left side of the forehead.

After the wounds had healed, it became obvious that the deformity of the donor site was almost as bad as the original deformity had been. The patient was understandably dissatisfied. A second operation was required to fill in the donor site defect, and this time methylmethacrolate was used.

This error obviously occurred because of inexperience, but it could have been predicted quite easily. When taking a bone graft from the skull, it would certainly make sense to take it from a part that is well-covered by hair so that the donor site defect is not visible.

## *23. The Case of the Missing Colostomy*

The patient was a 58-year-old man with cancer of the rectum. He underwent abdominoperineal resection, which proceeded uneventfully, though it took somewhat longer than usual as the surgeon took great pains to explain each step to the two medical students who were observing.

As the abdominal incision was being closed, the surgeon noticed that one of the students looked very puzzled.

Finally the student managed to bring himself to ask his question, which was, "How is the patient going to be able to manage his bowel movements?"

The surgeon, being a very patient man, explained that the patient would use his colostomy.

The student then looked even more puzzled and asked, "What colostomy, sir?"

At that point the surgeon realized he had forgotten, in fact, to make the colostomy, which then required reopening the abdomen for that purpose.

## *24. The Fragile Steroid-Treated Patient*

The patient was a 67-year-old woman with a long history of rheumatoid arthritis for which she had been treated with Prednisone. She was admitted to the hospital with a four-week history of gradual swelling on the side of her face, which was increasing and beginning to cause a great deal of pain. A diagnosis of parotid abscess was made and the patient was taken to the operating room for incision and drainage.

A small incision was made on the side of the cheek and a large collection of pus was encountered. There were some additional swollen areas above and below the site of the incision, and it was decided to try to drain these through the same incision. However, while the surgeon was manipulating a finger through the incision the skin tore, opening up a large wound almost the entire length of the cheek.

The lesson to be learned from this case is that an elderly patient with a long history of steroid therapy will have extremely weak connective tissues, and this fact also applies to the skin. The surgeon was extremely surprised by how little force it took to produce this injury, and will undoubtedly be more careful in manipulating a wound in this type of patient in the future.

## *25. "Almost" Only Counts in Horseshoes*

The patient was a 56-year-old businessman with a history of chronic intermittent claudication that had, over the past several weeks, progressed to rest pain in the right leg. Arteriograms demonstrated obstruction of the superficial femoral artery with reconstitution of the popliteal artery. Therefore, a femoral popliteal bypass was the planned treatment.

At operation, a saphenous vein graft was obtained and the common femoral artery and popliteal artery were exposed through standard surgical approaches. The proximal anastomosis was done first and the vein graft was passed through subcutaneous tunnels to the popliteal space, where it was found that the vein graft was about 2 centimeters too short to reach the popliteal artery. This required obtaining an additional vein graft and an additional anastomosis.

The lesson to be learned from this case is that it is better to make a vein graft a little too long than to make it a little too short. Trimming off the extra length from the vein graft is of no great consequence, but having a vein graft that is too short is a potential disaster.

The basic rule here is to measure twice and cut once. Remember that "almost" only counts in horseshoes. A near miss is fairly good in thermonuclear war but completely inadequate in vein grafting.

## TWO

# ERRORS IN JUDGMENT

GOOD JUDGMENT comes from experience, and experience comes from bad judgment. The most difficult aspect of surgery lies in choosing the right path. Here are some examples of surgeons who went the wrong way. It's easy to make an incorrect decision; the key to success is to recognize the error soon enough to correct it before any harm is done.

## *26. Fat People Are Different*

At about midnight, the junior resident called the chief resident to inform him that he had seen a patient in the emergency room with classical signs and symptoms of appendicitis.

In accordance with the normal procedure in that particular teaching hospital, the chief resident told the junior resident to go ahead with an appendectomy and to call him if there were any problems. The junior resident, however, neglected to mention that the patient was five feet tall and weighed 300 pounds.

After induction of anesthesia, the abdomen was prepped and the right lower quadrant was draped. A four-inch transverse incision was made in the right lower quadrant. The dissection was continued through the fat with the intention of entering the abdomen through a muscle-splitting incision.

As might be expected in a 300-pound patient of this stature, the abdominal fat was quite thick, and before long the deepest retractors were in place and the fascia had still not been identified. Deeper retractors were obtained and the dissection was continued down into the fat, but visibility was difficult because of the short incision and the depth of the wound. Eventually, a rather tough-looking structure was encountered and when this was incised and retracted, a green sheet was observed in the bottom of the wound.

At this point, the junior resident finally realized he had exceeded his capabilities and called the chief resident for help. The chief resident quickly solved the problem by extending the incision medially; he then located the external oblique fascia and completed an otherwise uneventful appendectomy.

Obviously, the initial incision went through the flank and exited through the patient's back. The problem could have been avoided if the junior resident had had a better appreciation of the anatomy of obese persons, but it could just as easily have been avoided by making an incision of adequate length. Wide people require a wider incision. Fortunately, there were no serious untoward effects from this surgical misadventure.

## *27. Don't Underestimate the Injury or Overestimate the Patient*

An 82-year-old man was brought to the hospital after sustaining burns that covered 15 percent of the total body surface area. When seen in the emergency room, he appeared to be in good condition with a second degree burn and stable vital signs. The resident considered sending the patient home and decided against it only because his home had burned down.

The patient was admitted to the surgical ward where he was given a regular diet, and routine vital signs were ordered. Over the next several days he deteriorated rapidly and developed infection in the burn wounds, which subsequently became full-thickness. At that point he was transferred to the burn unit. After a long and protracted course, the patient eventually died of his burn wounds.

The lesson in this case is that even a relatively small percentage second degree burn can be a lethal injury in older patients. The resident obviously both underestimated the severity of the injury and overestimated the recovery powers of the patient. A second degree burn of this size in a younger patient might well have been manageable on an outpatient basis. In an older patient, an injury of this type can be life threatening.

## *28. The High Velocity Gunshot Wound*

The surgeon had recently arrived in Viet Nam after completing surgical training in a county hospital that provided extensive experience in trauma.

His first patient was a young soldier who was brought in by helicopter a few minutes after having been wounded in action. On examination, the only abnormalities were a small entrance wound in the right flank near the mid-axillary line and what appeared to be an exit wound about 6 cm posterior to the entrance wound. The surgeon probed the tract between these two wounds and found that the bullet had passed subcutaneously.

He took his patient to the operating room, where he planned to open the skin between the two wounds and debride the subcutaneous tissue. However, a more experienced surgeon looked at the patient and suggested that the abdomen be explored. The primary surgeon was somewhat skeptical but elected to follow this advice.

On exploration of the abdomen he found that the right colon was completely necrotic from the cecum to the hepatic flexure. In addition, the right kidney had been completely shattered. He performed a right hemicolectomy and a right nephrectomy, and the patient made an uneventful recovery.

The lesson learned from this case is that a very high velocity missile, such as is found in military-type wounds, can produce a substantial amount of damage that may extend well beyond the actual path of the bullet.

## *29. It's Hard to Make an Asymptomatic Patient Better*

The patient was a 63-year-old man who previously had had an abdominal operation at another hospital many years ago. From the history it seemed there had been a postoperative wound infection, and when it had finally healed the patient developed a large midline incisional hernia. He was not particularly bothered by this hernia and had been managing the problem for many years with a corset.

He was now being seen by his physician for difficulties with shortness of breath, which on further workup proved to be due to chronic obstructive pulmonary disease. He also had chronic bronchitis. He had smoked two packs of cigarettes a day for many years.

In the course of his general examination the hernia was noted and he was referred to a surgeon. The surgeon advised a repair of the hernia and the patient agreed, only because he did not wish to refuse to take medical advice, and subsequently underwent ventral hernia repair in a standard manner.

Postoperatively, the patient developed respiratory failure requiring a mechanical ventilator, and later he developed signs of heart failure, followed by wound infection, systemic sepsis, and septic shock. The wound separated and eventually healed by secondary intention, leaving him with a large ventral hernia, much larger than the one he had originally.

After 30 days in the intensive care unit and an additional 30 days in a hospital room, the patient was able to return to his previous sedentary life and still seemed to manage his hernia quite well with an abdominal corset.

The moral of this story is that it is very difficult to make an asymptomatic patient better. It is not, however, very difficult to make an asymptomatic patient worse, particularly if he has significant concurrent disease.

## *30. The Case of the Accidental Impendectomy*

A 25-year-old man was admitted by way of the emergency room shortly after an autombile accident. He had findings of left upper quadrant tenderness and a dropping hematocrit, which was suggestive of blunt trauma to the abdomen. Because of these findings he was taken to the operating room for exploratory laparotomy.

On exploration, he was found to have a rupture of the spleen and a retroperitoneal hematoma that extended into the ileocolic mesentery. The spleen was removed. During the process of exploring the abdomen, his appendix was examined and was thought to be slightly deformed by what appeared to be an old scar. The surgeon elected to remove the appendix.

The patient's postoperative course was initially benign, but on the fifth postoperative day he began having high spiking fevers and increasing left upper quadrant pain. He developed a left pleural effusion and was noted to have poor excursion of the left hemidiaphragm. An ultrasound of the abdomen was suggestive of a fluid collection in the left upper quadrant. On re-exploration the patient was found to have a subphrenic abscess, which was drained. The patient went on to make a prolonged but successful recovery.

The subject of incidental appendectomy at the time of abdominal exploration is still a little controversial, but at the time of intra-abdominal injury requiring removal of traumatized tissue in a wound that is otherwise not contaminated, the wisdom of introducing a source of contamination is certainly subject to question.

Although an appendectomy in the absence of inflammation induces very little contamination, it is not unlikely that that was the source of the infection, and it greatly complicated this patient's course.

## *31. The Case of the Wrong Operation by the Wrong Surgeon*

A 22-year-old woman had a long history of well-documented ulcerative colitis. In spite of maximal medical therapy, she continued to be very symptomatic and was therefore referred to a surgeon. The patient was very well-educated on the subject of her disease and specifically requested to have an operation that would preserve the anal function.

The surgeon had had very little experience with ulcerative colitis, but he had heard of sphincter preserving operations and agreed to her request. He subsequently did a subtotal colectomy and brought the right colon through the pelvic floor and the anal sphincter as a pull-through. The patient made a very poor recovery, with persistent pelvic abscesses, and draining sinuses and fistulas about the perineum. She continued to lose weight and to have severe diarrhea.

Eventually she was referred to another surgeon, who treated her with a preoperative period of hyperalimentation followed by a total colectomy and ileostomy. Following that procedure the patient made a dramatic recovery and returned to a normal state of health.

There are a number of very fundamental and serious errors in the mangement of this patient. First and foremost, the primary surgeon did not recognize his own limitations. The surgical treatment of ulcerative colitis is total proctocolectomy, and that is a very well-accepted principle of the management of this disease. There are differences of opinion and differences in technique for the management of the ileum, including pull-through operations and continent ileostomies, but the safest and most conservative operation is the permanent ileostomy. The surgeon should have recognized that the sphincter-preserving operation was a relatively new concept and certainly one with which he was not familiar. The fact that he did not seem to realize that removal of the entire colon was essential to irradicate the disease was quite obvious from his choice of operation. These two deficiencies in his education should have prompted him to refer the patient to a surgeon who was more qualified to deal with her specific problem. At the very least, he should have taken the trouble to learn as much as possible about the management of this disease before undertaking such a difficult case.

All surgeons have their limitations and there is no shame in ignorance. The real shame is in not recognizing our ignorance, and either correcting it or getting the patient to someone who is more capable.

## *32. The Case of the Ignorant L.M.D.*

At about 7:00 P.M. on a Friday evening, a surgeon who was in private practice at a small community hospital called a major teaching hospital 50 miles away, asking to transfer a patient. He was referred to the resident on call.

He described the patient to the resident as having severe left lower quadrant pain and a tender left lower quadrant mass. He related to the resident that he was concerned because the small community hospital in which he practiced did not have an intensive care unit or a blood bank. The resident told the surgeon that this was clearly a case of diverticulitis and proceded to advise the surgeon on how to manage that disease, refusing to have the patient transferred because the problem was much too simple to be referred to a major medical center.

At about midnight the private surgeon called back and spoke to the same resident. He explained that the patient seemed to be getting worse and that his hematocrit had dropped and he was developing signs of shock. The resident then told the surgeon that the patient was too sick to transfer.

The referring physician was not particularly happy with this bind and managed to contact the resident's chief of surgery, who contacted the resident and arranged for the patient to be transferred. The chief of surgery then waited, expecting to hear from his resident after the patient arrived at the medical center. He heard nothing further about the case, but encountered the resident at a conference the next morning. At that time the resident told him the patient had indeed arrived, but was not as advertised: he was completely stable and not very sick.

After the conference was over, the resident and his chief

went up to the ward to see the patient. The more senior surgeon examined the patient and found a pulsatile left lower quadrant mass. The patient had a normal blood pressure, but gave a history of poorly controlled hypertension. The laboratory results from the tests ordered on admission revealed a hematocrit of 20. The patient was promptly taken to the operating room for repair of a ruptured iliac aneurysm. The resident was fired and subsequently returned to his native land.

The lessons to be learned from this case are obvious, but deserve emphasis. There is an endemic disease of the attitude that is, unfortunately, rather common among residents. The victims of this disease tend to assume that any referring physician who is not associated with a major medical center must somehow be unintelligent and inexperienced. The irony is that most of these residents will themselves be in private practice, many of them in small community hospitals with limited facilities. The second major area of error in this case is obviously that the resident evaluated the patient so poorly that he, himself, did not recognize the seriousness of the patient's condition.

## *33. Septic Phlebitis*

The patient was a 45-year-old man who was being treated on the medical service for systemic candidiasis, which apparently arose as a complication of his treatment for leukemia.

An intravenous line was placed in the cephalic vein just above the elbow, and Amphotericin was administered. The patient initially appeared to be responding well, but after several days, he developed a high fever and signs of shock. There was some inflammation over the course of his cephalic vein, and a surgical consultation was obtained.

The surgical resident made a correct diagnosis of septic phlebitis and took the patient to the operating room for excision of the vein. He made a long incision along the course of the vein and found it to be thrombosed, with a substantial inflammatory reaction around the vein. He excised the vein up to where it disappeared between the deltoid and pectoralis major muscles and transected the vein at that point. He noticed that there was still pus and thrombus in the remaining vein, but did not feel he could do any further excision himself. The wound was packed open and he obtained a thoracic surgery consult to see whether they felt they could do any further excision of the vein. They indicated to the surgical resident that they did not think that a central vein resection was feasible and, therefore, essentially nothing else was done. The patient died the following day.

This particular case indicated an unfortunate lack of knowledge and experience in the syndrome of septic phlebitis. Typically, the thrombosis and purulence in the vein will extend proximally until the major branch is reached. Had the resident resected the cephalic vein all the way to the axillary vein, it is most likely he could have completely eradicated at least this aspect of the patient's disease. He was obviously not thinking clearly in believing that he could not adequately expose this area, since a simple division of the pectoralis major insertion, as in radical mastectomy, would have provided ample exposure of the axillary vein. His assumption that the axillary vein would be involved in the septic thrombosis was almost certainly incorrect and he missed an opportunity to salvage a patient who might have gone on to some further reasonable quality of life.

## *34. Retained Common Duct Stone*

The patient was a 68-year-old man with a history of intermittent jaundice. A diagnosis of common duct obstruction from gallstones was made and confirmed with a transhepatic cholangiogram. On exploration, it was found that he had multiple stones in the gallbladder and a dilated common duct with palpable stones.

A cholecystectomy was done and the common duct was explored, with removal of several stones. However, on T-tube cholangiogram, it was apparent that a single large stone was lodged in the distal common duct. The stone appeared to be producing almost complete obstruction, as there was no flow of dye into the duodenum. Several attempts were made to retrieve this stone but all were unsuccessful; therefore the decision was made to put a T-tube in the common duct and close the patient, with a tentative plan to have a radiologist attempt to retrieve the stone at a later time. However, when the later time arrived, the radiologist was also unable to retrieve the stone. This left the patient with a large amount of bile draining from his T-tube and the usual problems of steatorrhea and malabsorption resulting from this abnormal diversion of bile.

Several significant errors in judgment were made in this case. In retrospect, it might have been wise to delay removing the gallbladder until it had been determined that the common duct could not be cleared. Since the cystic duct was patent, it would have been possible to divert the patient's bile with an anastomosis of gallbladder to small intestine, either duodenum or jejunum. Even if the gallbladder had not been retained, it would have been possible to do a diversion directly from the common duct to the duodenum or jejunum, since this was a large dilated common duct.

Even in those cases in which it is determined not feasible or safe to do an anastomosis of biliary tract to intestintal tract, significant problems can be avoided by placing a jejunostomy tube, allowing the T-tube from the common duct to be connected to the jejunostomy tube to allow reinfusion of the patient's bile.

In this case, the major advantage would have been the avoidance of a second operation, or gaining an interval that would have been far more healthy and comfortable for the patient. The decision to rely on the interventional radiologist to retrieve the stone at a later time was highly questionable since the radiologist would not have the advantages the surgeon had in direct manipulation of the common duct.

## *35. The Danger of Sigmoidoscopy Under Anesthesia*

The patient was a 32-year-old man who presented to his primary physician with a 3 centimeter inguinal mass. A biopsy was done, which showed the mass to be an enlarged lymph node containing malignant melanoma. The surgeon then did a careful search of the skin of the lower torso and extremity but found no sign of a primary melanoma, and the patient was unable to give any history of a previous suspicious lesion. It was decided, therefore, that the patient have a lymph node dissection.

Preoperatively, bowel cleansing was done with the intent of doing proctoscopy under the same anesthetic, to rule out the possibility of a rectal mucosal melanoma. The attending left the resident to do the proctoscopy at the end of the lymph node dissection. The resident subsequently reported to his attending that he saw no abnormalities in the lower bowel until he went beyond a 15 cm level. At that point he said he had considerable difficulty in making the turn of the sigmoid, and after several attempts managed to advance only a short distance. He then mentioned that the only abnormality he saw was what appeared to be a lipoma. The attending surgeon suddenly recognized that the resident most likely had perforated the bowel in trying to visualize the bowel proximal to the 15 cm level. A laparotomy was promptly done, with a finding of a perforation of the lower sigmoid colon. The perforation was repaired and, because the bowel had been prepped only with a single enema, a diverting sigmoid colostomy was deemed necessary.

This case represents a number of areas of questionable

judgment. In retrospect, there was not really much reason to do the proctoscopy under anesthesia instead of preoperatively. It is not unlikely that if there had, in fact, been a rectal mucosal melanoma, the plan of operation would have changed significantly.

Another error was in attempting to pass the sigmoidoscope beyond 15 cm, and this was an error for two reasons. First, it is extremely unlikely that the patient had melanoma beyond that point presenting as an inguinal lymph node metastasis. A simple rectal proctoscopy would most likely have been sufficient. Second, when the patient is under general anesthesia, the risk of perforating the bowel is increased significantly. Under anesthesia, it is much more difficult to turn the corner at the upper level, and the patient is unable to protect himself by complaining of pain.

Finally, the "lipoma" that the resident saw was epiploic fat, and it was indeed fortunate that his attending realized that before a delay in diagnosis resulted in peritonitis.

## *36. What Were You Going to Do About It Anyway?*

A 48-year-old alcoholic with cirrhosis and moderate portal hypertension was admitted with complaints of chronic right upper quadrant pain. He had reasonably good liver function and had never had any bleeding, although he did have some esophageal varices. On ultrasound examination, he was found to have stones in the gallbladder. A decision was made to do a cholecystectomy.

The dissection was difficult, and during the operation a considerable amount of bleeding was encountered from both the abdominal wall and the gallbladder. By the time the gallbladder was removed, the patient had required nine units of blood but was otherwise stable. Before closing the abdomen the common duct was palpated, and in the process of this examination a mass was felt in the head of the pancreas.

There was some concern about cancer of the pancreas, so it was elected to biopsy the mass. The biopsy showed only a focus of chronic pancreatitis. The patient, however, continued to bleed from the biopsy site in the pancreas, and the hemorrhage could not be controlled. Eventually, the patient was closed in spite of continued bleeding, and he subsequently died on the first postoperative day.

There are two significant errors in judgment in this case. In the first place, the patient had only moderate symptoms and was therefore not an ideal candidate for elective cholecystectomy in view of his known portal hypertension. The nine-unit blood loss during cholecystecomy should not have been unexpected since the portal hypertension could be expected to result in large dilated veins in the gallbladder and in the abdominal wall.

That error was dwarfed to insignificance by the error that was committed later. When the mass was felt in the head of the pancreas, it was certainly justifiable to consider the possible diagnosis of cancer of the pancreas. However, the surgeon neglected to give due consideration to what he would do about a cancer of the pancreas if, in fact, he proved one to be present. The patient was clearly not a candidate for resection, and therefore the results of the biopsy could be of prognostic and academic interest only. In view of what was to be gained from that biopsy, the price was indeed high.

## *37. Poor Planning in Vascular Surgery*

The patient was a 69-year-old man who presented with an ischemic ulcer of his right leg and pain in the leg at rest. He had multiple medical problems, including chronic obstructive pulmonary disease, chronic congestive heart failure, and a history of severe pancreatitis several years earlier that had required drainage of a pancreatic abscess. An aortogram demonstrated obstruction of the right common iliac artery and stenosis of the left common iliac artery. The right femoral artery was reconstituted by collaterals and the left femoral artery seemed to have good filling through the external iliac.

Because of the patient's poor medical condition it was elected to treat him with a femoral-femoral bypass, and this procedure was carried out uneventfully. However, in the early postoperative period it was noted that he had severe ischemic changes in his left leg. At that point a repeat arteriogram was obtained, and this time more distal views were taken, which showed that the femoral-femoral bypass was apparently filling the right lower extremity reasonably well, but that the left superficial femoral artery was obstructed and there was poor visualization of the popliteal artery. An emergency left femoral-popliteal bypass was considered, but the patient's ischemic changes rapidly progressed to gangrene, requiring amputation of the left leg.

The error made here was that of not obtaining an adequate workup before proceeding with reconstructive vascular surgery. Had the surgeon been aware of the more distal obstruction of the left femoral system, he most probably would not have selected the left femoral artery as the donor artery for revascularization of the right lower extremity. That could have been accomplished by more extensive arteriography, or perhaps more simply by measuring the ankle blood pressure. In retrospect, a right axillary-femoral bypass would have been a much better choice for this patient and almost certainly would have avoided or delayed the loss of his left leg.

## *38. The Case of the Aborted Abdominoperineal Resection*

The patient was a 68-year-old man who was admitted with a several-day history of lower bowel obstruction. It was readily apparent on rectal examination that he had a large tumor, and a biopsy confirmed adenocarcinoma of the rectum. It was determined by physical examination that the tumor was not resectable, and therefore he underwent a period of preoperative radiation therapy. The plan was to follow this with a palliative abdominoperineal resection.

At the time of laparotomy he was found to have metastatic cancer in the liver and a smaller primary tumor with extensive fibrosis in the pelvis. Several hours were spent trying to dissect out the distal sigmoid and rectum from the abdominal approach, but the tissue was very fibrotic and the tumor involvement was still significant. Ultimately, it was decided that the tumor was not resectable, and therefore an end sigmoid colostomy was done. The distal sigmoid was brought out as a mucous fistula.

During the postoperative period the mucosa of the mucous fistula was very dark, and over the next several days it gradually turned black. The patient developed a pelvic abscess that required open drainage. He spent an additional three months in the hospital before he was well enough to go home, and he lived another three months after that.

The error in this case was obviously one of judgment. The distal segment of bowel was devascularized before it was determined that it could not be removed. Once it had been determined that resection was not possible, the sigmoid colostomy was appropriate, but leaving the devascularized distal bowel in place probably contributed to the postoperative sepsis and morbidity. A better alternative may have been to resect as much of the distal segment as possible and close it as a Harman's pouch. A far better solution would have been to recognize the unresectability of the tumor before the colon was devascularized.

## *39. The Case of the Overtreated Cough*

A 41-year-old woman saw her family doctor because of a persistent cough. The doctor found nothing alarming on physical examination, but elected to have a chest X-ray done. The X-ray showed normal lungs, but the radiologist noted an apparent bone tumor in the right proximal humerus.

The patient was then referred to a major medical center for a thorough workup, including CT scan. On her initial physical examination, she was found to have a lump in her breast and it was elected to biopsy that first. The breast lump proved to be only a fibroadenoma, but the incision for the biopsy became infected, eventually resulting in an unsightly scar.

Results of the CT scan suggested that she probably had a benign cartilagenous tumor of bone, but it was believed desirable to confirm that with a biopsy. That biopsy confirmed that the tumor was, in fact, a benign cartilagenous tumor that required no treatment. Unfortunately, the wound incision in the arm also became infected, and, in addition, she developed a prolonged radial nerve paresis.

Somehow, during all these therapeutic misadventures, the patient's cough spontaneously resolved. However, she was treated for two other, asymptomatic, conditions, neither one of which would have been discovered had she not gone to her physician with a cough. She probably would have been much better off had they not been discovered.

This case once again illustrates the point that it is very difficult to make an asymptomatic patient better, but it is very easy to make one worse.

# THREE

# ERRORS IN MANAGEMENT

THIS CATEGORY of error is used to classify those that deal with the non-operative, non-technical aspects of patient care. Surgeons must be more than cutting technicians; they must also be doctors and practice medicine. In teaching hospitals this aspect of patient care is sometimes delegated to the least experienced member of the team. Even experienced surgeons can stumble in this category, so watch your step.

## *40. Iatrogenic Headache*

During the evening rounds, the chief resident suggested that the postoperative intestinal resection patient would benefit from intravenous hyperalimentation. The junior resident noted that on his list of chores.

By the time the junior resident returned to the patient to place the intravenous line, it was quite late in the evening. He did a standard subclavian vein puncture and advanced a catheter into what he presumed was a central vein. The X-ray technician was not immediately available, so the resident decided to initiate the hyperalimentation fluid and obtain an X-ray for catheter placement the next morning.

As soon as the infusion started, the patient complained of a severe headache localized in the left side. Not really knowing what was going on but suspecting it must have something to do with the infusion, the resident stopped the IV flow and the patient's headache immediately disappeared. Fascinated by this observation, the resident repeated the maneuver several times until he was certain it was the infusion that was causing the headache. At that point he decided perhaps he would get an X-ray after all.

The film showed the catheter had not passed centrally but had passed across the subclavian vein to the opposite side and had ascended the internal jugular vein. The tip of the catheter was lying just inside the skull. Repositioning of the catheter resulted in significant improvement in the patient's tolerance of the intravenous infusion.

The lesson to be learned from this experience is that there is really no substitute for following procedures, and an X-ray for catheter placement is mandatory before starting infusions of hypertonic solutions.

## *41. Remember the Chief Complaint*

A 45-year-old woman was brought to the emergency room by the paramedics after she had a grand mal seizure in the parking lot of a shopping center. Because she had no previous history of a seizure disorder, she was admitted to the medical service for a diagnostic workup.

After several days of intensive diagnostic tests, no cause for the seizures could be found. She was noted, however, to be moderately anemic, so additional studies were done to determine the cause of the anemia. During the course of these studies she was noted to have a positive stool guaiac. Consequently, a barium enema was ordered and this test proved to be normal; however, the scout film suggested the presence of gallstones, and therefore a cholecystogram was done, which confirmed the diagnosis of cholelithiasis.

She was transferred to the surgical service for treatment of her gallstone disease. Upon transfer, the physical examination was repeated, with the finding of a mass in the upper, outer quadrant of the right breast. On biopsy, this proved to be an intraductal carcinoma. A modified radical mastectomy was done, and two weeks later the patient underwent cholecystectomy with an uneventful postoperative course.

Seven days following that procedure the patient was discharged from the hospital and had a grand mal seizure on the way out the front door. It seems no one remembered she had originally been brought to the hospital because of a seizure disorder, and therefore the discharging physician neglected to continue her anticonvulsant.

The moral of this story is that it is always well to remember why the patient sought medical attention in the first place.

## *42. Watch Out for Drug Combinations*

A 34-year-old man had been diagnosed as having a gastrin secreting tumor, and for several weeks he had been managed with high doses of Cimetidine. But it gradually became apparent that his ulcer diathesis could not be controlled medically, and he was admitted to the hospital for operation.

After he arrived on the ward, the nurse called the resident, who was in the operating room, and asked for some preliminary orders. The nurse mentioned that the patient was extremely anxious and wondered if it would be all right to give him something for his nerves. The resident gave a telephone order for 10 mg of Valium to be given orally.

When the resident finished his operating room schedule for the day and went to examine the patient, he found him asleep, and he was unable to wake him. Upon reviewing the patient's chart, the mistake he made became quite apparent to the resident: the patient's high dose of Cimetidine was interfering with the metabolism of diazepam, greatly potentiating its effect.

The consequence of this error was that the resident had to wait until well after midnight before he could awaken the patient sufficiently to do his history and physical examination.

This case illustrates the importance of potential drug interactions. Cimetidine is notorious for interfering with the metabolism of certain drugs, such as diazepam, but also anticoagulants, Propanolol, and Antipyrine.

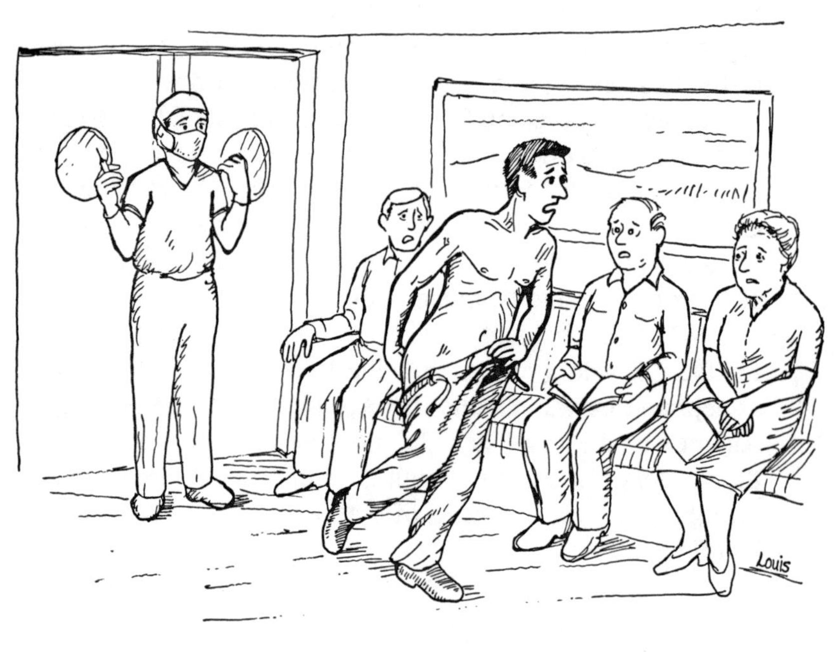
Louis

## *43. Loss of Patient Rapport*

A 35-year-old Mexican-American male came to the emergency room with a painful thrombosed hemorrhoid. He was seen initially by an intern, who consulted the surgical resident. The resident suggested incising the hemorrhoid under local anesthesia and removing the clot.

The intern neglected to mention that the patient spoke no English, and the resident neglected to adequately intruct the intern on the use of local anesthetics. Using hand signs, the intern managed to instruct the patient to assume a jack-knife position, after which he donned his gloves and, using a 20-gauge needle, he injected the hemorrhoid with 10 cc of Xylocaine.

The resident, who was three rooms down the hall, heard an ear-piercing scream and stepped into the hall to investigate. He was greeted with the sight of the patient running out of the treatment room, through a crowded waiting room, and out onto the street, still screaming at the top of his lungs, pulling up his pants with one hand, and holding his painful hemorrhoid with the other hand.

The intern was standing in the doorway of the treatment room still wearing his gloves and holding the offending syringe in one hand. As he watched his patient disappear down the street, he suddenly realized everyone in the waiting room was staring at him. He calmly looked about the room and said, "Next."

The lesson to be learned from this incident is that local anesthetics sometimes produce more pain than they relieve, and that a more appropriate method of administration would have been a very slow and gentle injection using a very small needle. The situation would have been helped immeasurably had the patient been warned to expect an injection.

These errors will certainly not be repeated by that particular individual. However, what he lacked in local anesthetic technique, he certainly made up in composure.

## *44. Pain Is the Best Narcotic Antagonist*

Late one night the intern was called to see a middle-aged man who had been admitted earlier that evening with a perirectal abscess. The patient had been started on antibiotics and was waiting for his turn to go to the operating room for incision and drainage. When the intern examined the patient, however, he found him to be quite toxic.

In checking with the operating room, the intern found that it would not be possible for the patient to go to surgery for several more hours. Therefore, he decided to drain the abscess in the surgical ward treatment room. The night nurse helped him put the patient on the treatment table and then went on about her duties in another room. The patient was obviously in a great deal of pain so the intern administered intravenous Demerol, even though the patient had already been receiving large doses of narcotics. A total of 200 mg was administered intravenously before the patient seemed comfortable enough to tolerate an injection of local anesthetic.

In spite of the local anesthetic and the large dose of Demerol, the patient remained very uncomfortable and experienced a great deal of pain when the incision was made and the pus was drained. Immediately afterward, the patient became profoundly comatose, with very shallow respiration, and gradually cyanotic. After a great deal of screaming and yelling, the intern was able to summon the nurse to bring a narcotic antagonist. However, he found he could stimulate the patient to breathe by pressing on the inflamed edges of the abscess. Subsequently, the narcotic overdose was reversed and the patient made an uneventful recovery.

The lessons to be learned from this case are first, a treatment room late at night without adequate help is a poor substitute for an operating room; second, local anesthesia is often inadequate for treatment of an abscess; third, and perhaps the most important lesson, a patient with a very painful lesion will have a tremendous resistance to narcotics. After the painful lesion is acutely corrected, this narcotic antagonist effect disappears and the patient then assumes the characteristics of an overdose patient. Fortunately, the intern had enough presence of mind to recognize this and was able to stimulate the patient to breathe by recreating the pain until a more definitive treatment could be administered.

## *45. Paraplegics Are Different*

A 25-year-old paraplegic man was transferring from his wheelchair to a car when he fell and sustained a fracture of his right tibia and fibula just below the mid-shaft. He was taken to a nearby emergency room where the fracture was reduced and a long-leg cast was applied.

About two weeks after the application of the cast, a foul odor was noticed, and a brown stain was seen over the lateral malleolus. When the cast was removed, a 6 cm pressure sore was found over the lateral malleolus with full-thickness loss of skin down to bone.

The primary lesson to be learned from this case is that paraplegics have a different set of priorities. The absence of sensation in the lower extremities precludes detection of a point of excessive pressure within a cast. The value of a long-leg cast is additionally suspect in that prompt solid healing of a tibial fracture in a paraplegic is of minimal value.

This problem could have been avoided by using external fixation in the mangement of the fracture. An equally rational approach to an injury of this type would have been to immobilize the extremity using two large pillows wrapped firmly around the extremity from the knee to the toes. This almost always leads to a fibrous union, but even a pseudarthrosis of the tibia in a paraplegic is of minimal, if any, consequence.

## *46. The Wrong Side*

A 24-year-old man with a history of spontaneous pneumothorax returned to the hospital with complaints suggesting another collapse of his lung.

The resident sent the patient to the X-ray department for a chest film. After the patient returned to the emergency department, the resident went down to X-ray to review the film, and noted that the patient had a left-sided pneumothorax.

The resident then returned to the emergency room, where he was interrupted by several more-urgent problems. It was at least an hour before he was ready to put in the chest tube. Then, he very carefully and skillfully introduced the chest tube into the right chest, but he did not detect any sudden rush of air as the chest tube was put on suction. When he sent the patient back for the post-thoracostomy X-ray, his mistake became quite obvious, as he saw the pneumothorax still present in the left chest and the chest tube in the right chest.

There are numerous examples, in all surgical departments, of cases in which the left and right sides have been confused. There are stories of incisions that have been made on the wrong side, operations on the wrong side for hernia, and even amputations of the wrong extremity.

All these mistakes can be avoided if one merely thinks about the possibility of operating on the wrong side.

In the case of the misplaced chest tube, the mistake could have been easily avoided had the chest X-ray been present in the room at the time the chest tube was inserted.

## *47. The Mysterious Drop in Blood Pressure*

A 42-year-old woman was admitted for elective cholecystectomy. The patient's history was typical for chronic cholecystitis. Before admission to the hospital, she had had an ultrasound study that showed multiple stones in the gallbladder.

On a thorough review of systems, the patient's only other complaint was that she had been troubled for several years with arthritis in her hands. Her family doctor had been treating her with pills, but the patient was not aware of the name of these pills and did not bring them to the hospital with her. On physical examination, there were no abnormalities other than mild obesity and a scar from an appendectomy many years before.

The patient's cholecystectomy was uneventful. In the recovery room she was noted to have low blood pressure of only 70/40. There was some concern about the possibility of bleeding within the abdomen, but the postoperative hematocrit was normal and follow-up hematocrits did not show any drop. She was given a bolus of Ringer's solution, which increased her blood pressure moderately, but she continued to be hypotensive throughout the night.

The next morning, after the intern had spent a sleepless night trying to control the patient's low blood pressure, the patient asked him when she could start taking her arthritis pills again. This prompted the intern to investigate further by calling the family physician, which is how he discovered that the patient had been taking Prednisone for several months. Administration of hydrocortisone promptly restored the patient's blood pressure to normal. Over the next several days she was tapered back to a maintenance dose and went on to recovery uneventfully.

The lesson to be learned in this case is that a thorough and accurate drug history is always important, and that any time a patient is being treated for arthritis or a related condition, the possibility of corticosteroids should be considered. If it is not possible to rule out steroid ingestion, it might be the better part of valor to go ahead and treat the patient with a bolus of hydrocortisone during the time of operation, which can then be tapered rapidly during the postoperative period. This will probably not harm the patient who does not have adrenal suppression, and might prevent disaster in one who does.

## *48. The Case of the Obstructed Colostomy*

This particular error occurred on three separate occasions in the same institution, about one year apart. It illustrates the principle that those who cannot remember history are condemned to repeat it.

All three events involved patients who had had a previous loop colostomy and, for various reasons, in each case it was deemed advisable to convert this loop colostomy into a complete diverting colostomy by closing the distal orifice with staples. In all three cases the wrong orifice was obstructed and, as you might guess, the error was extremely obvious about three days later.

Fortunately, there were no great consequences to these errors in that the functioning lumen was easily re-opened and the defunctionalized lumen closed. However, it is likely that if the surgeons had thought more about the possibility of obstructing the wrong lumen, they could easily have prevented the problem by passing the catheter up from below or some similar maneuver to avoid this mistake.

## *49. The Case of the Untreated Bowel Obstruction*

The patient was a 58-year-old man who came to the hospital complaining of abdominal distention and constipation. This problem had developed quite gradually, but was now becoming distressing to the patient. He was also having intermittent abdominal pain.

He was examined by the resident, who suspected a bowel obstruction, and this suspicion was further supported by the abdominal X-ray, which showed an extremely dilated transverse colon. A barium enema demonstrated a constricting lesion in the left colon with approximately 90 percent obstruction. The patient was then sent home to await elective admission for left colon resection for cancer.

He returned the following day with signs of peritonitis. He was explored immediately and was found to have a perforation of the colon just above the obstructing carcinoma.

The error in this case is quite obvious: the surgeon underestimated the severity of the patient's disease. Obviously, bowel obstruction requires more prompt and efficient management than was done here. The resident's decision to delay surgery in order to proceed electively was based on his desire to obtain a complete bowel prep; however, complete bowel prep would have been almost certainly impossible in the presence of the high-grade obstruction.

A more appropriate approach would have been to either do a temporary proximal colostomy or proceed with resection and end colostomy. Either approach certainly would have required a second stage closure of the colostomy, but would have been preferable to perforation, peritonitis, and sepsis.

## *50. Beauty Is Only Skin Deep but Ugly Goes All the Way to the Bone*

A 65-year-old man was severely debilitated from lower extremity atherosclerotic vascular disease. He had had a previous amputation of his left leg above the knee, and although he had a satisfactory prosthesis, most of his time was spent in a wheelchair because of claudication in his right leg.

One day, while sitting in his wheelchair, he spilled hot coffee on himself, burning the skin of the anterior distal leg. His primary physician treated him for three weeks, but the patient showed no signs of healing. He was then referred to a surgeon, who debrided the wound and covered the defect with a split thickness skin graft. In spite of ischemia of the leg the skin graft took well. However, on the third postoperative day the patient was noted to have complete necrosis of the skin of the posterior heel. This resulted in an infection and osteomyelitis of the calcaneus, and ultimately required a below-the-knee amputation.

In retrospect, this problem was obviously due to inadequate protection of the heel. All debilitated elderly patients at bedrest should probably have extra padding to protect the heel, but this is especially true of patients with peripheral vascular disease.

This tragic complication converted a relatively difficult burn problem into an impossible decubitus problem. It once again illustrates the importance of attention to seemingly minor details of postoperative care.

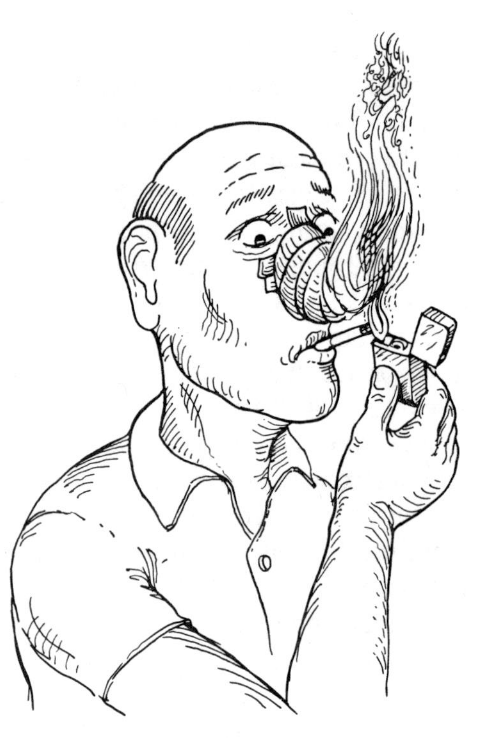

## *51. The Case of the Spontaneous Nasal Combustion*

The patient was a 62-year-old man who was admitted to a veterans hospital for treatment of extensive rhinophyma. After excision of the hypertrophic sebaceous nasal skin, a lot of blood kept oozing from the surface, so the surgeon applied a large bulky dressing.

Two hours later the surgeon received a frantic phone call from the ward nurse, who advised him that the patient's nose was on fire. The surgeon issued an immediate verbal order for extinguishment of the conflagration and went directly to the ward to investigate. There, he found the patient with a charred but soaking wet dressing, and when it was removed, he was greatly relieved to find that there had been no injury to the underlying skin.

In retrospect, this accident was quite predictable had the surgeon stopped to think about the peculiarities of the Veterans Administration patient population. The vast majority of these patients are compulsive cigarette smokers. On further questioning of the patient and the other men in the same ward, it became clear that as soon as the patient got back to his room and had access to his personal effects, he immediately got out a cigarette and flicked his Bic, igniting the nasal bandage.

The same sort of accident could happen with a nasogastric tube. Fortunately, there were no serious consequences to this particular incident.

## *52. The Dangerous Associated Condition*

The patient was a 75-year-old man who was admitted to the vascular service for symptoms of severe ischemia of the lower extremities. He was worked up with arteriograms, and a decision was made to do an elective aortobifemoral bypass. A review of his history revealed that he had had two previous attempts at hiatal hernia repair with only modest success.

The patient's operative course was relatively uneventful, and, according to the custom of the attending surgeon, the patient was given systemic heparin. However, postoperatively, the patient developed a massive upper gastrointestinal hemorrhage, which proved on endoscopy to be coming from a severe hemorrhagic esophagitis. Although the heparin was reversed and the hemorrhage was eventually controlled, the patient suffered a significant setback and had a prolonged recovery involving multiple system failure.

Retrospective questioning of the patient about his preoperative symptoms revealed that he still had frequent episodes of esophagitis, required frequent use of antacids, and slept with the head of his bed elevated. These persisting symptoms had been overlooked on the initial workup.

In retrospect, more awareness of the patient's preoperative symptoms of esophagitis might have allowed the surgeons to avoid the major complication. A realization that the patient was still fairly symptomatic from his esophagitis might have influenced the decision to use systemic heparin, but in any case would have mandated fairly close attention to prophylaxis, including frequent administration of antacids and elevation of the head of the bed.

## *53. The Management of Delirium Tremens Without Drugs*

The patient was an elderly alcoholic who had been admitted to the hospital for treatment of an abscess in his leg.

The treatment of his leg was progressing nicely, but on the fourth day in the hospital he developed a fairly clear-cut case of delirium tremens. The most distressing part of his delirium was that he was having hallucinations about snakes and was constantly wrestling with an imaginary snake that was trying to bite him. The intern treated the patient with ever-increasing doses of sedatives. The patient did not respond to this treatment and continued to wrestle with the imaginary snake.

The intern was becoming very concerned because he was afraid the patient would become exhausted. He called the chief resident who solved the problem quickly and simply by tying the imaginary snake to the bed rail with an imaginary rope. The patient immediately relaxed, thanked the doctors profusely, and went off to sleep.

The lesson in this story is that sometimes there are ways to treat problems other than with drugs.

# FOUR

# ERRORS IN DIAGNOSIS

SOME OF THE diagnostic errors in this section were due to the subtle nature of the patient's disease or injury, but most were a result of missing the obvious.

Surgeons are not usually thought of as diagnosticians, but no surgical procedure can be expected to succeed if it is based on an incorrect diagnosis. The surgeons who blindly accept the referring physicians' diagnoses do so at their own and their patients' peril. The easiest way to overlook the obvious is to not think of it. Sometimes this happens because the surgeon does not think at all. It is easy to be in a hurry and skip through the "routine" history and physical.

In the practice of surgery, time is often an expensive commodity, but time can be your best tool. Take time to listen to your patient. Take time to examine your patient. As the great Yogi Berra once said, "You can observe a lot by just looking."

## *54. Do the History and Physical Before the Operation*

A 23-year-old woman was referred for a mass in the right upper arm. The mass was described as firm and apparently attached to the upper end of the biceps muscle.

A routine X-ray was not revealing, but a CT scan demonstrated a radiolucent mass with poorly defined borders located in the upper medial arm near the origin of the biceps tendons. Based on the physical examination and CT findings, a tentative diagnosis of a sarcoma was made, and the patient was scheduled for an open biopsy and possible forequarter amputation.

During the dissection into the arm, a fibrous mass was encountered. When this was incised, a viscus, sticky fluid was encountered. Biopsies of the wall of the fibrous mass were consistent with scar.

The following day, as an afterthought, a careful history and physical examination were done. The patient then volunteered a history of having had an augmentation mammoplasty the year before. This was complicated by fibrous capsule contracture on the right side, which had been treated on an outpatient basis by her private physician, who did a closed capsulotomy. The patient related that the doctor had had to use a great deal of force to break the scar capsule, and, subsequently, she had had some pain in her shoulder and noticed her right breast was slightly smaller. It was about three weeks after the capsulotomy that she first noticed the lump in her upper arm. On physical examination, the patient had small axillary scars bilaterally, and the left breast was definitely larger than the right. Obviously, the implant had ruptured and some of the silicone gel was extruded into the axilla.

This case clearly indicates the importance of careful history and physical examination. Although no harm was done in this particular case, it is clearly preferable to do the work-up before the operation.

## *55. The Shortest Distance Between Two Points Is Not Necessarily a Straight Line*

The patient was a 52-year-old female, brought to the emergency room soon after sustaining a small calibre bullet wound to the left side of the neck. On her initial examination, she was in no distress and had no apparent hematoma in the neck. There was an entrance wound at the lateral edge of the left sternocleidomastoid muscle 3 cm above the clavicle, and the bullet was palpable in the subcutaneous tissue on the left side of the posterior neck, 4 cm lateral to the midline. Her vital signs and neurological examination were normal. On gastrographin swallow, there were no abnormalities in the esophagus and the bullet was readily visible in the posterior subcutaneous tissue.

The patient was taken to the operating room where under sedation and local anesthesia, esophagoscopy and bronchoscopy revealed no abnormalities. By the time the endoscopies had been completed, the patient was two hours post-injury and still had no hematoma in the neck. Since it appeared the wound was lateral to the great vessels of the neck, it was elected to observe her rather than explore the wound. She was transferred to a hospital room, and on the following morning she was found to be quadriplegic.

Further study of the neck film showed the bullet had traversed the vertebral body of C-5. A second film, after the quadriplegia was diagnosed, showed the vertebral body had collapsed, probably while the patient was being moved from the operating room to her hospital room.

The lesson to be learned from this case is that the bullet had obviously not traveled in a straight line from the entrance wound to its final location in the posterior neck. This is often the case when a bullet strikes bone, but it is even possible for bullets to be deflected by soft tissue. It is unlikely this disaster would have been prevented by an exploration of the neck. Since the X-ray findings were very subtle, perhaps only a very acute awareness of the possibility of deflection of the bullet by a bone would have led to the observation that the bullet had injured the vertebral body.

## *56. The Case of the Medical Surgeon*

A 48-year-old woman was admitted with classical signs and symptoms of acute appendicitis. She had a history of insulin dependent diabetes, but had been very stable on insulin management.

At the time of appendectomy, the patient was noted to have perforation of the tip of the appendix and a moderate amount of exudate in the right lower quadrant.

Postoperatively, her condition initially improved and in general she seemed to be doing fairly well, but then her diabetes became difficult to manage. The surgical housestaff, in their frustration, requested a medical consultation for help with the diabetes. The medical resident examined the patient, and on rectal examination he found a fluctuant mass. As he probed the mass, his finger pushed through into a pelvic abscess, which began draining into the rectum. The patient's diabetes promptly came under control, and her embarrassed but better educated surgeons discharged her three days later.

The lesson to be learned from this case is that difficulty with diabetes control can be the first sign of infection. Control of the infection can result in control of the diabetes.

## *57. Not Quite End-Stage Heart Disease*

A 6-year-old girl, who had been under treatment her entire life for problems related to congenital heart disease, had an endocardial cushion defect that required mitral valve replacement. This was done with a St. Jude mechanical valve.

She seemed to do well for quite some time, and then developed rapidly progessing heart failure and, in spite of maximal medical therapy, began deteriorating rapidly. The family was advised that the child had reached an end-stage phase of her disease and nothing more could be done.

The operating surgeon was advised of the patient's deteriorating condition and came around to see her and speak to the family. More to assure the family than for any other purpose, the surgeon listened to the child's heart. He was somewhat surprised that he could not hear the mechanical valve. On questioning, the mother related that she had stopped hearing the valve just a short time before the child began to rapidly deteriorate. The patient was promptly returned to the operating room where the valve was replaced. Examination of the defective valve showed the leaflets had been stuck in the open position.

The error in this case was in not recognizing the cause of the sudden deterioration and assuming it was a progression of the disease, which was known to have a very poor prognosis. If a more detailed history had been taken, the problem might have been suspected, but it should have been apparent from the lack of a mechanical heart valve sound on chest auscultation.

## *58. Don't Believe Anything You Hear and Only Half of What You See*

The patient was a 74-year-old man who was admitted to the medical service with upper gastrointestinal hemorrhage. During the first 24 hours after admission, he required six units of transfusion, and a medical consultation was requested.

On upper gastrointestinal endoscopy by the medical service, a modest amount of blood in the stomach was seen, but no mucosal abnormalities were noted. The duodenum was visualized and a large clot on the posterior wall could be seen, with blood coming out from under it.

This was assumed to be a duodenal ulcer. Because the patient had lost six units of blood, a decision was made to do a vagotomy and pyloroplasty. The patient was taken to the operating room for this purpose and the vagotomy was done first, through his midline laparotomy. A pyloroplasty incision was then made, and, on inspection of the posterior wall of the duodenum, no ulcer was found. Retractors were placed in the pyloroplasty incision and the stomach was inspected with some difficulty. It was then suspected that the patient had gastritis, although the abnormalities of the mucosa were not thought to be particularly dramatic. The pyloroplasty was completed and the patient was returned to the intensive care unit.

He continued to bleed and, on further investigation, was found to have a proximal gastric ulcer, which subsequently required gastrectomy.

There are two lessons that can be learned from this error in diagnosis. One is that endoscopy is not necessarily a definitive examination. In this case it led to an incorrect diagnosis, perhaps because of the relative lack of experience of the endoscopist.

The second lesson is that a more appropriate order of operation might have been to open the pylorus first, before doing the vagotomy. There are two reasons for this. First, the primary goal was to stop the bleeding — best done by direct exposure of the ulcer and suture ligation — and the secondary goal was to correct the ulcer disease, since it was the hemorrhage that was life threatening, not the ulcer itself. The second reason for this suggested order of operative procedure is that (as, in fact, it was in this case) the diagnosis might be incorrect, which would make vagotomy inappropriate.

A correct diagnosis might have been obtained in the operating room had better exposure been obtained by doing a more proximal gastrotomy. But it should be clear that the error in diagnosis led to an inappropriate operation. Consequently, the patient needed the correct operation at a later time.

## *59. The Case of the Constipating Carcinoma*

A 72-year-old man had been confined to a nursing home for several years because of senility. He was brought to the emergency room because of distention of his abdomen.

It was reported that he was chronically constipated, requiring frequent use of enemas and laxatives. On examination, he had a very distended abdomen and seemed to be tender in the left upper quadrant. The plain X-ray of the abdomen showed a massively distended loop of colon in the left upper quadrant, and, after consultation with the radiologist, a tentative diagnosis of volvulus of the cecum was made. Because the dimensions of the cecum were measured to be at least 17 cm on the X-ray, it was decided that he urgently needed decompression.

At operation, a small right transverse abdominal incision was made, and the torsion of the cecum was gently reduced. A catheter was introduced into the cecum to relieve the distention. The cecum was carefully sutured to the right lower quadrant, then the catheter was brought through the skin and placed on low, intermittent suction.

A few days later the patient seemed to be having reasonably normal bowel movements and his abdomen was flat and non-tender. He was placed on a regular diet and the cecostomy catheter was removed, but he continued to have fecal drainage from the catheter tract. After this continued for several more days, the problem was investigated with a barium enema, which demonstrated a constricting carcinoma in the descending colon. The patient later underwent a left hemicolectomy.

This case illustrates the danger of accepting the admission diagnosis as a final diagnosis. The surgeons were correct in their initial diagnosis of a torsion of the cecum, but failed to give due consideration to the possible underlying causes that might have led to the problem in the first place. Fortunately, the diagnosis was eventually established and the patient received appropriate treatment.

## *60. Sometimes the Sound of Hoofbeats Indicates Approaching Zebras*

### Case #1

The patient was a 58-year-old man who was seen initially in the emergency room with a history of having been stabbed in the abdomen with an ice pick.

He was hospitalized for observation and appeared to be doing well for the first two days, but then developed upper gastrointestinal bleeding. On abdominal examination, he had no signs of peritonitis. A technetium scan was done, which indicated that the bleeding was coming from the stomach or duodenum.

On gastroduodenal endoscopy, the source of bleeding could not be definitely identified, but he did seem to have edema in the first portion of the duodenum. A tentative diagnosis of peptic ulcer disease was made. The patient was taken to the operating room, where vagotomy and pyloroplasty were done, but again the source of bleeding was not positively identified.

The patient appeared to do well for two days, and then his bleeding recurred. This time an arteriogram was done, which indicated the bleeding was actually coming from the jejunum. On re-exploration, the bleeding site was identified in the jejunum: it was a traumatic arteriovenous fistula that was presumably a result of the stab wounds.

The error in diagnosis was apparently due to an inadequate workup and some unjustified assumptions. The technetium scan was obviously misleading and the endoscopy was overinterpreted. The arteriovenous malformation was missed because that possibility was not adequately considered. Fortunately, the patient did well following a small bowel resection.

## *61. Sometimes the Sound of Hoofbeats Indicates Approaching Zebras*

### Case #2

The patient was a 48-year-old man who was admitted with lower intestinal bleeding. Because he seemed to be bleeding actively, a technesium scan was done, which indicated the blood was coming from the right side of the colon.

The patient had lost enough blood to require transfusion with six units; therefore it was decided to remove the right colon for a presumed diagnosis of diverticulosis. However, pathologic examination of the specimen did not show any abnormalities. The next day the patient was noted to have continued bleeding. This time an arteriogram was done, which demonstrated bleeding from the distal ileum; on re-operation this proved to be from an arteriovenous malformation that was presumably congenital in origin. Resection of this lesion resolved the problem.

This error came from the assumption that the bleeding was coming from the colon, which was most likely because bleeding from the lower small bowel is very rare. The technesium scan was relatively nonspecific and misled the surgeon into believing that the source of the bleeding must be from the right colon. Later, an arteriogram proved to be more definitive, and established the correct diagnosis.

The lesson here seems to be that sometimes the most common possible diagnosis is not, in fact, the correct diagnosis.

## *62. The Acute Medical Abdomen*

The patient was a 54-year-old woman with Crohn's disease that had been partially controlled for many years with Prednisone, who now required surgery for a stricture of the colon. She therefore underwent resection of the stricture and re-anastomosis. At the same time, a fistula between the colon and small bowel was resected, requiring a small bowel anastomosis.

From the time of her operation, the patient was maintained on intravenous doses of cortisone, which was being gradually decreased. On the fifth postoperative day she was started on oral liquids and 20 mg of Prednisone by mouth per day.

The patient did well for the first four postoperative days. On the sixth postoperative day, she developed severe abdominal pain and a rigid abdomen. Her white count and serum electrolytes were normal. Her temperature was 38.5 degrees centigrade. She was returned emergently to the operating room, where the abdomen was re-explored. Although the preoperative diagnosis for the re-exploration procedure had been a leaking anastomosis and peritonitis, on exploration there were no signs of peritonitis and the bowel anastomoses were both intact.

As she was returned to the operating room she was again given an intravenous dose of cortisone, and this was continued postoperatively. The patient made a prompt recovery and ultimately left the hospital in good condition.

Obviously, the diagnosis of acute abdomen and disruption of bowel anastomoses had been incorrect. The far more likely explanation for her symptoms was adrenal insufficiency, which is known to produce physical signs indistinguishable from those of an acute surgical abdomen. In all probability the patient did not absorb the Prednisone when it was given orally because of residual bowel dysfunction and malabsorption.

Perhaps the best lesson to be learned from this case is that in patients with significant bowel disease, the surgeon should be cautious when switching from parenteral to enteral administration of steroids.

## *63. Sepsis in the Burn Patient Does Not Always Come from the Burn Wound*

A 78-year-old man was admitted to the burn unit with thermal burns covering 60 percent of the total body surface area. Because the wounds were largely partial thickness, they were treated with topical silver sulfadiazine. His initial resuscitation was successful. General supportive measures were used, which, because of poor dietary intake, included intravenous hyperalimentation.

On the tenth postburn day, the patient began having signs of sepsis, with some deterioration in the appearance of the wounds and a decrease in blood pressure. It was felt that he needed intensive monitoring with a Swan-Ganz catheter, but attempts at percutaneous placement of the catheter were unsuccessful. Therefore, a cut-down was done on the basilic vein and, after considerable difficulty, the catheter was successfully placed in the pulmonary artery.

The patient initially stabilized, but two days later he began a rapid deterioration with increasing signs of sepsis and a falling blood pressure. Sepsis in the cut-down site was suspected, and the Swan-Ganz catheter was removed and replaced with another catheter, which was placed percutaneously in the subclavian vein. The patient failed to improve, and in fact, continued his rapid deterioration. Inspection of the cut-down site showed what appeared to be only superficial infection. Later that day the patient was seen by a more experienced member of the team, who suggested exploration of the cut-down site. The incision was extended proximally and the entire length of the vein was removed. Within hours after the removal of the infected vein the patient demonstrated a dramatic improvement and went on to make a complete recovery.

An analysis of this case shows that perhaps two significant errors were made. In retrospect, the use of a cut-down for venous catheterization in a patient with a heavily colonized burn wound was ill-advised because of the high risk of contamination of the vascular system. The error was then compounded by failure to recognize the presence of a septic thrombophlebitis. Because of the patient's age and his large burn wound, it was assumed that the sepsis was due to deterioration of the wound. The possibility of septic phlebitis was not recognized until it was suggested by a more senior member of the team. If the problem had not been recognized and promptly corrected, it would certainly have resulted in the death of this patient.

## *64. The Case of the Wandering Bullet*

A 22-year-old man was brought to the emergency room after having been shot in a domestic disturbance. He had an entrance wound just above the right eye, and no exit wound was found. His physical examination was otherwise normal. A skull X-ray was ordered and a neurosurgeon was called.

The X-ray and the neurosurgeon arrived simultaneously. When it became apparent that the bullet had not entered the cranium, the neurosurgeon immediately lost interest and left the emergency room. On careful inspection of the X-ray, small fragments of the bullet were seen tracking down into the neck, but the bullet itself was still not visible. Therefore, an X-ray of the neck was ordered and an ENT resident was called.

The ENT resident and the new X-ray appeared simultaneously in the emergency room. The bullet was found to be not present in the neck, although there were continuing tracks of metallic fragments extending toward the chest. The neck examination was normal and the ENT resident lost interest and left the emergency room. A chest X-ray was ordered and the thoracic surgeon was called.

The thoracic surgeon and the chest X-ray arrived in the emergency room at approximately the same time, and this time the bullet was found. It appeared to be at approximately the level of the diaphragm on the left side. There was no evidence of hemothorax or pneumothorax, therefore the thoracic surgeon also lost interest. But before leaving the emergency room he suggested calling the general surgeon because he thought the bullet was probably below the diaphragm.

The general surgeon did not agree that the bullet was below the diaphragm, and he also expressed a somewhat limited interest since the patient's abdominal examination was normal. However, with there being no further services to which the patient could be passed on, he felt compelled to admit the patient for further observation. The following morning the intern obtained another X-ray and this time the bullet was seen in the mid-abdomen. The abdominal examination was still normal, so it was elected to continue observation. The following day another X-ray was taken and the bullet was gone. The patient's examination was still normal and he was observed for another three days and was then discharged.

It is quite obvious, in retrospect, that the bullet had penetrated the enteric tract at some point. Three possibilities immediately come to mind. The bullet may have passed through the chest and the diaphragm and entered either the stomach or the transverse colon. Anatomically, the stomach would seem more likely, but the rapid passage through the GI tract would suggest the possibility of an entrance directly into the colon. However, the complete lack of abnormal physical findings on abdominal examination seemed to rule out those possibilities. In addition, the chest X-ray never showed any evidence of any pulmonary abnormalities, making it seem unlikely that the bullet had passed through the entire length of the lung. A third possibility is that the bullet entered the pharynx or cervical esophagus and was passed through the GI tract from that level.

This case does not necessarily represent an error. However, it does illustrate a relative lack of awareness on the part of the surgeons involved, and also the potential peculiar behavior of bullets.

## *65. Sometimes Small Injuries Are Not as Small as They Look*

A 30-year-old man came to the emergency room after sustaining injuries in an altercation at a local drinking establishment. He was noted to be moderately intoxicated. His nose was broken and he had a small laceration of the right hand over the dorsal aspect of the middle finger metacarpophalangeal joint. Treatment consisted of reduction of his nasal fracture and application of a nasal splint. There was no treatment given for his apparently minor hand injury.

Three days later the patient returned to the emergency room with massive swelling of his right hand and exquisite pain over the middle finger metacarpal-phalangeal joint. The laceration was draining a small amount of pus.

He was taken to the operating room where the hand was explored. A septic arthritis of the MP joint was found, with early destructive changes in the articular cartilage. The joint was drained and a splint was applied. He was hospitalized for seven days on intravenous antibiotics. Subsequently, he continued to have considerable stiffness of the entire hand with only 20 degrees of active motion in the involved joint, and limited motion in the other MP joints. With six months of intensive occupational therapy, he gradually regained satisfactory hand function.

The lesson to be learned from this case is that the original hand injury was obviously underestimated. A laceration over the MP joint of the dominant hand with a history of a fist fight almost always indicates that the laceration was produced by a tooth. An injury of this type must always be considered to be a human bite, and a strong possibility of penetration of the joint must also be taken into consideration.

The appropriate management would have been to take the patient to the operating room primarily for exploration of the wound, and possible drainage and irrigation of the joint. That should be followed by application of a splint and several days of intravenous antibiotics. Although this might have seemed to be overtreatment of an apparently minor injury, the consequences of missing a contaminated penetrating wound in a joint are well-illustrated by this case.

Another important point to be learned from this case is that when engaging in fist fights, it is best not to hit your intended victim in the mouth, and perhaps it is best to hit him with something other than your hand.

## *66. Remember the Thyroid*

A 45-year-old executive consulted a plastic surgeon for correction of baggy lower eyelids. When relating his history, he explained that he had recently begun to feel the onset of middle age and believed he was not as competitive in the business world as he had been in the past. He thought that some improvement in his appearance might be helpful. A thorough history was taken and revealed only non-specific complaints, such as easy fatiguability and chronic constipation, both of which the patient attributed to age. He was scheduled for lower eyelid blepharoplasty as an outpatient.

When the patient arrived at the outpatient surgical center, he was given the routine premedications, which at that facility were 10 mg of intramuscular diazepam and 50 mg of intramuscular Demerol, and was placed on a stretcher. Within 15 minutes the nurse noted that he had depressed ventilation and appeared to be cyanotic. She found that his blood pressure had dropped to 90/50, and immediately summoned the surgeon. The surgeon placed the patient on oxygen, reversed the narcotic, and had the patient admitted to the hospital. Needless to say, the operation was canceled.

A medical consultation was then obtained. The consultant felt that on the basis of the history, the patient might have hypothyroidism. This diagnosis was confirmed by laboratory studies and the patient was started on thyroid medication. During the subsequent weeks, the patient's general condition improved dramatically and the bagginess of his lower eyelids disappeared entirely.

There are two important lessons to be learned from this case. The first is that in hypothyroid patients, edema of the lower eyelids can be readily corrected by administration of thyroid hormone; moreover, the pills do not leave any scars. The second lesson is that hypothyroid patients are extremely sensitive to narcotics and the surgeon was indeed fortunate that the consequences were not greater than they were.

## *67. The Case of the Pseudo-Burn*

A 22-year-old woman was brought to the emergency room after having been found in her apartment in a stuporous condition. She was unable to give any history, but she had an obvious problem in the upper extremities. The ambulance attendants left without providing any other information to the doctor.

On examination, the patient had red blistered skin of both upper extremities from the elbows to the mid-palm. A tentative diagnosis of burn injury was made and the patient was placed in appropriate burn dressings and transferred to the burn unit. After 24 hours in the burn unit, she became more alert, and on questioning it became apparent that she was unaware of having been involved in any fire.

Further investigation revealed that the patient had, in fact, been found lying prone with both forearms and hands folded under her chest on a hard floor. Eventually, it was learned that she was addicted to narcotics, which made it apparent she actually had had a pressure injury to the upper extremities. The patient was taken directly to the operating room where forearm and hand fasciotomies were done, which showed compressed necrotic muscle. She subsequently went on to develop all the classic signs of a Volkman's contracture.

The consequences of this error in diagnosis were tragic in that permanent loss of upper extremity function might have been prevented if the diagnosis had been made promptly, and if decompression had been done at an appropriate time. Perhaps the error could have been avoided by an earlier and more thorough investigation of the patient's history — the diagnosis of a pressure injury might have been suspected had the physicians been more aware of that possibility.

## *68. Things Aren't Always What They Seem*

A 25-year-old alcoholic sustained a gunshot wound to the abdomen during a barroom brawl.

At laparotomy he was found to have penetration of the large and small bowel and of the pancreas. The small bowel was repaired and a colostomy was done. His postoperative course was complicated by sepsis and pancreatitis. He developed respiratory failure and a tracheostomy was subsequently performed.

On the eighth postoperative day the physician was called by the intensive care unit nurse and advised that the patient was becoming belligerent and was attempting to pull out his intravenous lines and his tracheostomy cannula. All attempts to communicate and reason with him were unsuccessful. Restraints were applied and the patient was given sedation.

The following morning the patient was seen by a more experienced physician who promptly recognized that the patient was hypoxic and removed the tracheostomy cannula. The patient immediately became calm and relaxed. Examination of the tracheostomy cannula showed that it was almost completely occluded by a mucus plug. A new tracheostomy cannula was inserted, and the patient went on to make an uneventful recovery.

An analysis of this error shows that a patient was assumed to be in delirium tremens because of his alcoholism and his uncontrollable behavior. The first physician failed to make the diagnosis of hypoxia because he did not consider that possibility.

## *69. The Case of the Cancer-Induced Hernia*

The patient was a 48-year-old heavy-equipment operator who was referred to a surgeon for treatment of an inguinal hernia. He underwent a routine hernia repair and recovered promptly.

One year later he returned to his physician with complaints of increasing constipation that could no longer be controlled with normal laxatives. A review of his history showed that he had, in fact, began having increasing diffculties with constipation during the month prior to developing the hernia. Further diagnostic workup demonstrated a partially obstructing carcinoma of the sigmoid colon, for which a sigmoid resection was done.

This case illustrates once again the important principle of taking a careful history in all patients, even those who seem to have fairly obvious and routine problems. In retrospect, it is clear the patient's inguinal hernia was at least in part related to his acquired bowel obstruction, in that the bowel problem caused straining that either caused or aggravated the hernia. Had the surgeon been alert to this possibility at the time he performed the initial hernia repair, he may well have been able to make the diagnosis one year earlier.

## *70. The Case of the Traumatic Ulcer*

A 52-year-old businessman was brought to the emergency room after an automobile accident. He was complaining of severe abdominal pain.

On physical examination, his vital signs were stable and he was found to have multiple contusions and abrasions about the face. Palpation of the abdomen revealed board-like rigidity and extreme tenderness. An upright chest X-ray showed free air under the diaphragm. A tentative diagnosis of blunt rupture of the jejunum was made.

On exploration of the abdomen, however, the patient was found to have a perforated duodenal ulcer. This was treated in the usual manner. Postoperatively, further discussion with the patient indicated he had a long history of peptic ulcer symptoms, and the accident occurred when he was driving to work and had a severe pain in the abdomen, causing him to let go of the steering wheel.

This case represents an error in preoperative diagnosis that had no therapeutic consequence, but once again illustrates the importance of an accurate pre-op history.

## *71. The Case of the Undiagnosed Headache*

The patient was 14-year-old boy who had been to his pediatrician with complaints of a headache. The pediatrician was sufficiently impressed that he obtained a CT scan of the head, which was somewhat equivocal but was thought to be suspicious for a posterior fossa mass.

Consequently, a transfemoral carotid arteriogram was obtained, and this ruled out the presence of an intracranial tumor. However, during the arteriogram the patient had an acute onset of severe left flank pain. A surgical consultation was obtained because the radiologist was concerned that he may have injured the aorta and produced a retroperitoneal hemorrhage.

The examining surgeon was impressed with the patient's flank pain and obtained a urinalysis, which showed hematuria. It was thought that the patient might have a renal artery injury or perhaps even a renal infarction. Consequently, it was decided to do a repeat arteriogram to examine the renal vessels.

The second arteriogram demonstrated a segmental renal artery obstruction and an apparent infarction of part of the kidney. During the arteriogram the patient developed severe hypertension, which required the administration of Nitroprusside for control of his blood pressure. On closer inspection of the arteriogram, the patient was noted to have a tumor blush just above the right kidney. Subsequent workup confirmed the diagnosis of pheochromocytoma of the right adrenal gland.

In retrospect, although the patient had been noted to have borderline hypertension, the significance of this was completely overlooked until the second arteriogram. There had been multiple opportunities to have made this diagnosis at an earlier time, but the problem was that no one thought of it. The surgeon and the radiologist both suffered from tunnel vision; each had been consulted for a specific problem and each failed to review the entire diagnostic picture. Fortunately, the patient suffered no ill effects from the delay in diagnosis and was subsequently successfully treated for his pheochromocytoma. He required no treatment for the partial infarction of his left kidney.

## *72. The Case of the Incomplete Physical*

The patient was a 21-year-old university student who was seen at the university infirmary with vague complaints of abdominal pain. After seeing two different physicians at the infirmary on two separate occasions, he was finally referred to the medical service of a nearby teaching hospital.

There, he was given a fairly extensive evaluation by the medical service, including multiple abdominal contrast studies and computerized tomography. It was determined he had a retroperitoneal mass and was referred to the surgical service.

On the surgical service, he was seen by several surgeons, but no physical abnormalities were noted and the retroperitoneal mass was not palpable. The patient underwent exploratory laparotomy, and a biopsy of the mass was obtained, which returned a diagnosis of metastatic testicular tumor.

It was not until that time that the patient had an adequate examination of his testes, which showed a very obvious tumor that could not have been overlooked if anyone had thought to check.

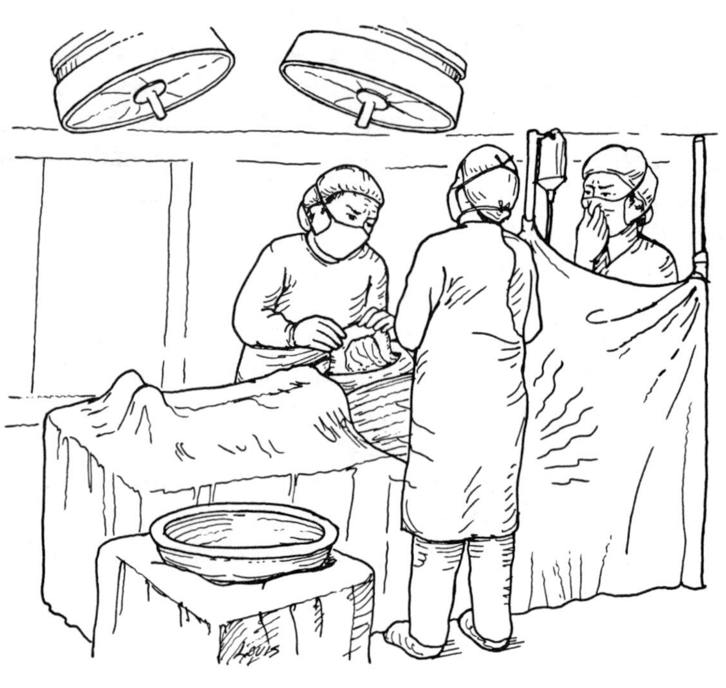

## *73. Who Fired That Shot?*

A 45-year-old man underwent an operation for intestinal obstruction. The cause of the obstruction appeared to be adhesions from previous abdominal surgery, and the lysis of adhesions required to correct the obstruction was prolonged and difficult.

After sufficient adhesions had been released to relieve the obstruction, the surgeon spent a considerable time searching up and down the bowel, meticulously examining every aspect of it. After this had been going on for some time, the assistant, who had not worked with this particular surgeon before, became curious as to why the surgeon was spending so long examining the bowel. The surgeon explained that he was looking for a perforation and he was sure that there must be one because he smelled bowel gas. The assistant was too embarrassed to explain that he himself was the source of the bowel gas and was the unfortunate victim of the previous evening's dinner at a local Mexican restaurant.

I suppose the lesson to be learned by this one is that before you spend a lot of time searching for a leak, you might try to tactfully inquire into the status of the other people at the operating table. Fortunately, the consequences of this error were minimal and consisted only of a modest increase in operating time.

## *74. The Benign Tattoo*

The patient was a 47-year-old woman who had had a mastectomy for cancer of the breast. She had also received postopertive radiation therapy.

On routine follow-up she seemed to be doing well, but the resident noted several small pigmented lesions near the border of the radiation field. He was concerned about the possibility of a radiation-induced melanoma and obtained punch biopsies of each of the pigmented spots. The following week he received the pathology report, which was "intradermal pigment and foreign body reaction consistent with tattoo."

What the resident had been looking at were the permanent markings for the radiation field, which some radiation therapists make with tattoo ink. Fortunately, there was no harm done by this little error other than a minor bruise to the resident's ego.

## *75. Tunnel Vision*

The patient was a 45-year-old alcoholic with a history of chronic pancreatitis, which had been managed by his internist for the past several years. Eight years ago, he was referred to a surgeon for peptic ulcer disease, and he underwent vagotomy and pyloroplasty.

As time went on, the chronic pancreatitis continued to get worse and the patient developed mild diabetes and pancreatic exocrine insufficiency. His diarrhea, which had been controlled with pancreatic enzyme replacement until fairly recently, was getting worse to the point he was having six to eight stools a day and had lost 30 pounds. In addition, during this same time the abdominal pain was also becoming gradually worse.

He again sought care from the surgeon for relief of these symptoms. The surgeon performed an endoscopic retrograde cholangiopancreatography, which confirmed partial obstruction of the pancreatic duct and showed a normal biliary tract. The patient was then explored with a plan of a decompression of the pancreatic duct with a Roux-Y. However, on exploration, the stomach was found firmly adherent to the transverse colon and when it was dissected free, it was found that the patient had a perforation of his stomach into the colon. At that point it became clear that the cause of his diarrhea was, in fact, a gastrocolic fistula, presumably on the basis of peptic ulcer disease.

Because the surgeons were not prepared to do a colon anastomosis, a colostomy was necessary. The stomach was repaired. The patient later underwent closure of his colostomy. These two procedures relieved his symptoms, which were evidently not due to the pancreatitis at all but related entirely to his gastrocolic fistula.

The error in this case was in assuming that the original disease was producing the new symptoms. A more thorough workup with an open mind would probably have led to the correct diagnosis and made it possible to avoid the need for a colostomy.

In retrospect, had a more careful inspection of the stomach been done during his endoscopic pancreatography, the diagnosis could have been made at that time.

## *76. The Case of the Irreparable Nerve*

The patient was a 55-year-old man who had been in an automobile accident. His only significant injury was a major laceration of the cheek that extended into the parotid gland. He was found to have a complete facial paralysis on the involved side.

The importance of nerve repair was emphasized to the patient, and, therefore, instead of repairing the wound in the emergency room under local anesthesia, he was taken to the major operating room and given a general anesthetic. Exploration of the facial nerve required removal of the superficial lobe of the parotid gland. When the entire area had been explored, no laceration could be found in any part of the nerve.

The next day the surgeon profusely apologized to the patient for being unable to find and repair the nerve injury. The patient did not seem to be particularly upset by this news and, in fact, consoled the surgeon.

"That's okay, doc. It's been paralyzed like that ever since I had a stroke five years ago, and I'm kind of used to it now."

The lesson in this case should be obvious. Even when you think the diagnosis is apparent, it is still a good idea to take a history.

## FIVE

# ERRORS IN COMMUNICATION

THE ERRORS REPORTED in this section could easily be classified in one of the other categories. I have separated them out to make a point. People — patients or colleagues — do not always understand what we say, or misinterpret the message. Be aware of the possibility and perhaps you can avoid one of those embarrassing moments in the practice of surgery.

## *77. The Case of the Recurring Gallstones*

The patient was a 45-year-old woman who had a long history of intermittent right upper quadrant pain that was associated with nausea and vomiting and fatty food intolerance. Because of this history, an oral cholecystogram was obtained, and this showed multiple small filling defects in the gallbladder. The patient underwent an elective cholecystectomy, which was uneventful.

Three days following the operation she told her surgeon she would like to be able to keep her gallstones. The surgeon, responding to her request, called the pathologist, who said he had no objection and would bring them around to her room later that day.

When the pathologist arrived on the ward, the patient was on the bedpan, and, not wishing to disturb her, he gave the student nurse the small plastic cup containing the gallstones and told her, "Give these to the lady in room 523." The student nurse did not happen to be acquainted with the pathologist. She looked into the container and saw a large number of small pearly-white objects. When the patient was finished using the bedpan, the student nurse took these to her and had her swallow them. The mistake was discovered the following day when the patient once again asked for her gallstones.

This case is not really an error in surgical management but rather an error in pathological and nursing management, or perhaps, to be more accurate, an error in pathological nursing management. Fortunately, the stones passed harmlessly and the patient really had no grounds for complaint since she asked for her gallstones, and had, in fact, received them.

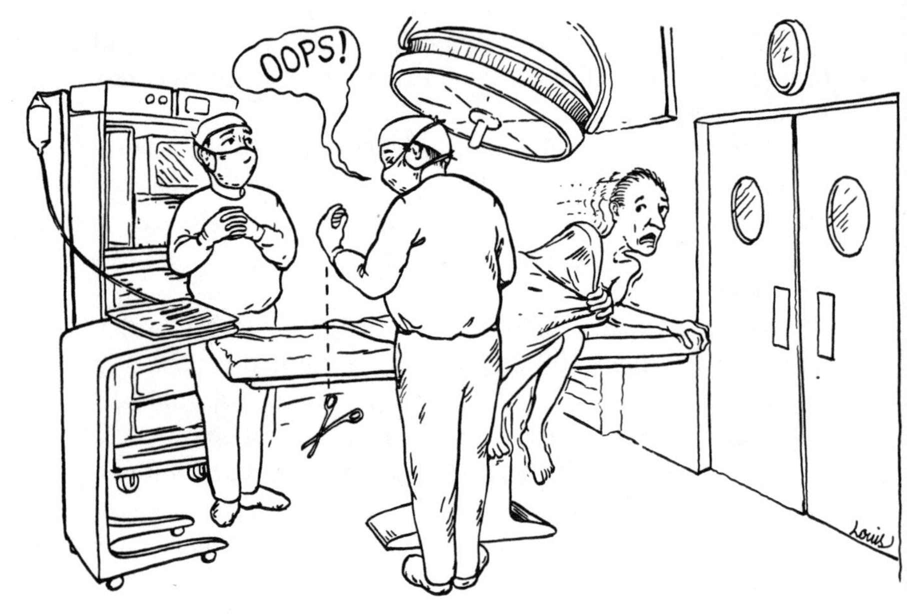
OOPS!
Louis

## *78. Never Say Oops!*

The patient was a 23-year-old man with a long history of paraphimosis. On the advice of his physician, he somewhat reluctantly agreed to undergo circumcision. This was to be done under local anesthesia, and the patient was brought to the minor surgery suite, where routine prepping and draping was done. Of course, after the drape was in place, the entire patient was covered except for the penis, which was left protruding through an opening in the sheet. Xylocaine was infiltrated until adequate anesthesia was obtained.

While the instruments were being prepared, the surgeon dropped an instrument on the floor, and said

"Oops!"

As it turned out, that was all the patient needed to hear. He came off the table like he had been shot out of a cannon. He wrapped the drapes around himself and stormed out of the operating room.

The intern was sent after the patient for the purpose of trying to persuade him to return to the operating room. He eventually found the man standing in the hall, still wrapped in a green sheet, apparently unaware that his still-anesthetized penis was hanging out of the hole in the drape. At this point it was very clear all rapport had been lost, so the operation was cancelled.

The moral of this story is, obviously, to always watch what you say. Anything an anxious patient overhears is subject to misintepretation. When using local anesthesia, never, never say oops!

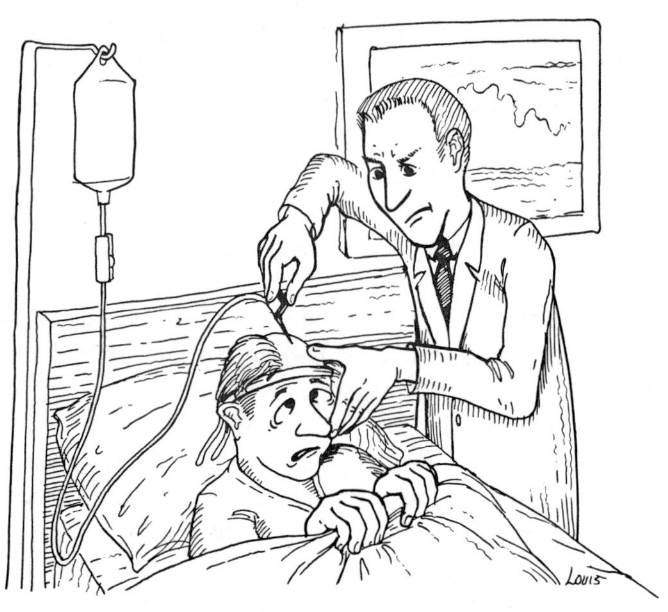
LOUIS

## *79. Sometimes Students Are Even More Stupid Than They Look*

Shortly after morning rounds on a busy surgical service, the nurse informed the resident that a patient down the hall needed a new IV. The patient was a 45-year-old man who had undergone gastric surgery two days earlier, and it was anticipated he would need IV fluids for one or two more days.

The resident then sent the medical student to start the IV line and told him to "use a 19-gauge scalp vein," meaning a butterfly-type needle. He neglected to consider that this was the student's first day on the service and that his only previous rotation had been on the pediatric service.

When the student did not return after about one hour, the resident became concerned and went down the hall to investigate. He found that the student had shaved the man's head, had placed a large rubber band around the head, and was trying for the fifteenth time to insert a butterfly needle into a vein in the scalp. The use of scalp veins for intravenous access is a common and accepted practice in the management of infants, but it is not generally thought to be a good method for adults.

The student should have been able to figure this out for himself, but the resident should have given more consideration to the limited experience of this student before sending him off to do a task.

## *80. You'd Be Amazed at What People Worry About*

The resident had just completed a routine hernia repair and, knowing the patient's family was waiting, he went by the ward to tell them the operation had been completed safely.

He was greeted by a large family, all of whom looked quite concerned. The patient's son acted as spokesman for the family.

"Well, how was everything, Doc?"

"Everything was just fine. We fixed his hernia and he should be able to go home in a few days."

"Well, I mean was everything really okay?"

"Sure, everything was fine. It was just a hernia."

"Well, are you sure everything will be okay, Doc?"

At this point the resident's supervising attending, who had been overhearing the conversation, stepped up and said,

"There was no cancer."

"Oh, thank God!"

The entire family appeared to be enormously relieved and all left the waiting room together.

The moral of this story is that most lay people do not really have any idea what a hernia is, and the general public has a natural and understandable fear of cancer.

## *81. Make Sure You Have the Right Person*

### Case #1

At about 3:00 in the morning the intern was awakened by the intensive care unit nurse. She told him the blood that had been cross-matched for Jose Gonzalez had finally arrived, and would he please come to start the transfusion.

The intern, who was still not quite awake, got out of bed and came down to the intensive care unit. He found that the nurse was busy with another patient, but the unit of blood was there on the table and was already connected to an intravenous administration set. He checked the name on the bag of blood, then took it over to Mr. Gonzalez' bed and hung the bag on the IV pole.

As he was running the blood down the tubing to expel all the air, he glanced across the room and noticed that the name tag of the patient in the next bed also said Jose Gonzalez.

Suddenly he woke up a little more, and remembered he had not requested any blood to be cross-matched for his patient. He decided it might be a good idea to check the hospital number on the blood and on the patient's identification bracelet. Noting they did not match, he took the blood down from the IV stand and delivered it to the correct Mr. Jose Gonzalez.

In this case the catastrophe was avoided, but the potential consequences are obvious.

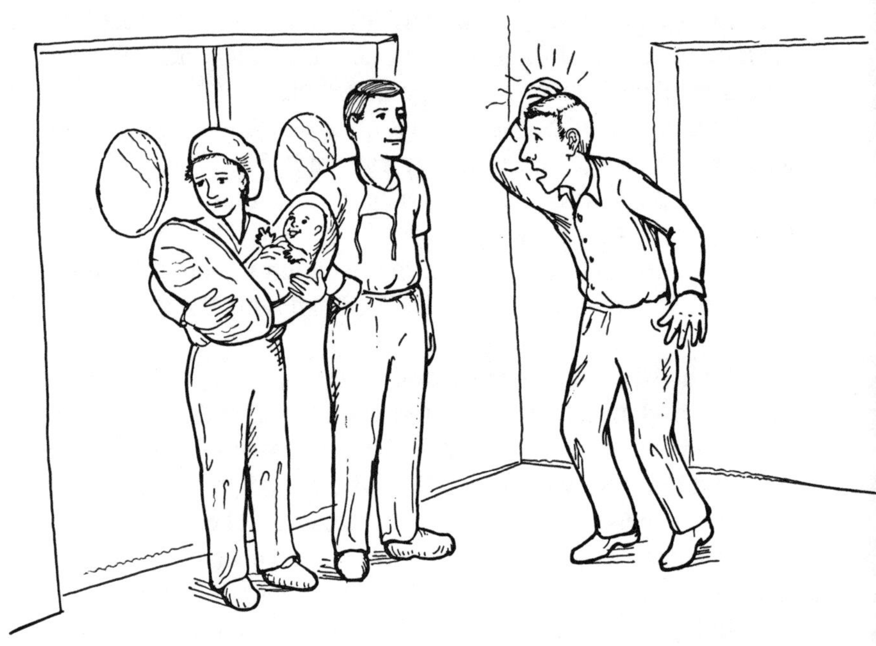

## *82. Make Sure You Have the Right Person*

Case #2

The obstetrical resident had just finished a difficult caesarean section, delivering twins. As he was finishing the procedure he noticed the general surgeons bringing a female patient into the room next door.

He changed his clothes and left the operating room. A rather worried-looking gentleman was standing outside the door.

"Are you waiting for Mrs. Hubbard?" the resident asked.

"Yes, I am. I'm her husband," he replied.

"Well, we just finished her operation and everything is fine."

"Really, that's amazing."

"Congratulations! You have twin boys and they're both fine. Your wife is doing fine, too."

"What!!!"

"I said your wife had twin boys and she and the babies are doing just fine."

At this point the man became visibly shaken and pale and had to sit down.

"But the doctors downstairs said they thought it was appendicitis."

As the conversation went on, it became apparent to the resident that the patient he had seen brought into the operating room was also named Mrs. Hubbard.

Fortunately, the second Mrs. Hubbard underwent an uneventful appendectomy and both she and her husband made a satisfactory recovery.

## *83. Make Sure You Have the Right Person*

### Case #3

An elderly gentleman with advanced cancer was failing rapidly, and the resident, knowing the patient was Catholic, called the chaplain. He gave the chaplain the patient's name and room number on 3rd East.

The chaplain, unfortunately, had a poor sense of direction. He went to 3rd West, where, in the room with a corresponding number, he encounterd a patient with the same name. However, the patient in 3rd West was in the hospital for an elective hernia repair the following day.

After being thoroughly consoled by the chaplain and given last rites, the hernia patient decided not to have his operation after all.

This error, of course, is not a surgical error, but an error in ecclesiastical management, and once again emphasizes the dangers of mistaken identity.

## *84. Students Aren't Always as Stupid as They Look*

The patient was a three-year-old girl with a large hemangioma of the neck. She was admitted for elective resection of this tumor and underwent routine history and physical examination and laboratory studies. As was the practice at that institution at that time, the complete blood count and differential count were done by the medical students.

The evening before surgery, the student assigned to her case reported to the resident that the hematocrit, white blood count, and differential count were normal, but that when he did the blood smear he was unable to find any platelets. The resident, who at that moment was busy writing orders in the chart, murmured an acknowledgement and went on with what he was doing.

The following morning the patient was taken to the operating room, and while the anesthesia was being induced, the student mentioned to the attending surgeon that he had not seen any platelets when he did the blood smear and wondered if that didn't have some significance. The attending surgeon appeared somewhat alarmed by that news and immediately cancelled the operation, returning the patient to the ward where a later study by the laboratory confirmed the diagnosis of thrombocytopenia.

The resident in this case made the error, perhaps because he had not given adequate thought to the possibility of thrombocytopenia, which is one of the potential consequences of a large hemangioma. He compounded this error by not really listening to the medical student and assuming the medical student merely failed to perform the blood smear properly. Significant consequences were avoided when the appropriate information reached a more experienced physician.

## 85. *The Case of the Sleepwalking Surgeon*

A 35-year-old man had been involved in an automobile accident and was admitted to a large teaching hospital with signs of an acute abdomen and a dropping hematocrit. At exploratory laparotomy he was found to have a laceration of the right lobe of the liver with some active bleeding; this was controlled with large sutures. He was returned to the intensive care unit in stable condition.

It was the custom in this hospital for the chief resident to be responsible for the patients on his service 24 hours a day, regardless of the call schedule. Therefore, even though the chief resident had been up all night operating on trauma cases, including this patient, another emergency necessitated his spending the following night in the operating room. The next day he still had a busy elective schedule, and by the end of that day he had been without sleep for approximately 56 hours.

While making afternoon rounds, the intern reported to the chief resident that the patient with the liver laceration had been requiring a unit of blood every two to three hours, his abdomen was becoming distended, and there was blood coming from the drains. The chief resident seemed to be listening attentively; he nodded his head and told the intern to continue giving transfusions. He then went home and went to sleep.

The next morning on rounds it was reported that the patient had received ten units of blood during the night and now the abdomen was massively distended. It was quite obvious to the chief resident, as it should have been the night before, that the patient had intra-abdominal hemorrhage. He gave the intern a severe tongue lashing for not having recognized this obvious problem and demanded to know why he had continued to give transfusions without informing the senior staff of the problem. The intern defended himself by reminding the chief resident that he had, in fact, informed him of the problem the evening before on rounds.

In this case the blame must rest with a system that allows the chief resident to work beyond his physical capacity. Nevertheless, the intern should have recognized that the chief resident was not functioning mentally and he should have taken the problem to another member of the staff.

Fortunately, the problem was managed successfully by re-operation, and the patient made an uneventful recovery.

## *86. The Case of the Thirsty Snake*

The patient was a middle-aged woman who previously had had multiple abdominal operations and one enterolysis for bowel obstruction.

She was being seen for another episode of bowel obstruction requiring enterolysis. During the operation the surgeon passed a long intestinal tube well into the jejunum to help decompress the bowel. The tube was placed on suction and the patient was returned to the floor.

During the subsequent two days she recovered her peristalsis very nicely. The tube began advancing farther down the intestinal tract. Nevertheless, the surgeons elected to keep the tube on suction since she still seemed to be somewhat distended.

The following morning, they entered the room on rounds and found the patient sitting on the bedpan with a look of absolute terror on her face. When they inquired as to what was troubling her, she explained that she had just urinated into the bedpan and a red snake had come out of her rectum and drank all the urine.

The surgeons were somewhat skeptical at first, but rolled her over and took a look; sure enough, there was the intestinal tube that had passed all the way through. This problem was easily corrected by some reassurance and removal of the tube.

## *87. But You Didn't Say Which Half*

The patient was an obese 50-year-old man who had undergone a ventral hernia repair and had been discharged from the hospital with his sutures still in place.

He returned to the clinic ten days after the operation. The wound did not appear to be sufficiently healed to remove all the sutures, so the resident asked the student to remove half the sutures, and then left the room to see another patient. A few minutes later the student came to report that the wound had opened, and he wanted further instructions as to what to do next.

When the resident went to take a look, he found the student had not understood that he was to remove alternating sutures, and had instead removed the upper half of the sutures.

## SIX

# HAZARDS OF MODERN TECHNOLOGY

MODERN MEDICAL EQUIPMENT HAS MADE possible many of the advances in surgical care. But some of these devices are complex, and subject to mechanical failure. And sometimes the surgeon is not adequately familiar with the operational characteristics or potential dangers of a given medical device. It is not unusual for a surgeon to begin using a piece of new equipment without reading the instruction manual. Sometimes a new technique entails risks that are not even recognized by the profession as a whole.

## *88. The Dangers of Equipment Failure*

### Case #1

The patient was a 22-year-old man with a fracture of the fifth metacarpal. When he was seen initially in the emergency room, the fracture was reduced and a short-arm cast was applied, but when he was rechecked three days later, the volar angulation of the distal metacarpal fragment had recurred and was considered significant. Therefore, the patient was advised to have a closed reduction and pin fixation.

It was elected to use an intravenous regional anesthetic, and the procedure was done in a sterile manner in the cast room. After the hand had been thoroughly prepped, a tourniquet was applied to the upper arm. A plastic catheter was inserted in a vein on the dorsum of the hand. The hand was then elevated long enough for the veins to empty and the tourniquet was inflated to 250 Torr; 50 cc of 1% Lidocaine was injected into the peripheral vein and the catheter was removed. The fracture was reduced and closed. When it appeared to be in a suitable position, percutaneous Kirschner wires were used to immobilize the fracture in its reduced position.

While waiting for the postreduction X-ray, the patient became extremely cyanotic and started having generalized seizure activity. Fortunately, there was resuscitation equipment handy, and the patient was given oxygen and ventilated with difficulty. As the seizure began to subside, an endotracheal tube was inserted and the patient was given 100 percent oxygen, which resulted in a considerable improvement in his skin color. An intravenous line was started in the uninjured extermity, and the seizures were finally brought under control with intravenous pentobarbitol. It was at that point it was found that the tourniquet had deflated. Apparently the problem was a defective cuff.

This case illustrates one of the major hazards of intravenous regional anesthesia. While 500 mg of Xylocaine is a safe dose when infiltrated subcutaneously, it is a highly toxic dose if administered by an intravenous bolus. Normally, with an intravenous regional anesthetic, the Lidocaine is confined within the extremity by the tourniquet and there is no systemic absorption as long as the tourniquet is inflated. After a few minutes the drug becomes fixed to the tissues, and by half an hour after administration, it is safe to deflate the tourniquet.

The errors made in this case were, first, that the equipment was obviously defective and was not adequately tested prior to its use. Second, the physicians were not adequately prepared for such an emergency: they did not have a separate intravenous line established prior to the incident. It is possible that if the cause of the seizures had been recognized more promptly, some benefit might have been achieved by reinflating the tourniquet.

The major error involved a lack of appreciation of the potential danger of the intravenous regional technique and the lack of appropriate preparation.

## *89. The Dangers of Equipment Failure*

### Case #2

The patient was a 45-year-old woman who had a severe laceration of the volar side of her wrist, caused by broken glass when a window she was replacing broke in her hand. She had multiple tendon lacerations and a laceration of the median nerve.

These injuries were repaired under general anesthesia using a tourniquet on the upper arm. The surgical procedure was uneventful and the patient was discharged the following day without any complications having been noted.

Her hand and forearm were in a splint and her arm was in a sling for several days. When seen in follow-up with the splint removed, it was noted that the patient had no active wrist extension and, in addition, she had apparent paralysis and anesthesia in the ulnar nerve distribution, even though the ulnar and radial nerves had not been lacerated.

Further investigation resulted in the discovery that the tourniquet used in the operation was seriously out of calibration and probably, instead of delivering 250 Torr pressure during the operation, had, in fact, delivered pressure in excess of 500 Torr.

This case illustrates the importance of careful maintenance of operating room equipment. This is particularly true of pneumatic tourniquets; it is generally considered advisable to check the calibration of a pneumatic tourniquet at regular intervals when in use, ideally at least once a day. Fortunately, the patient eventually recovered full function in this upper extremity, but this type injury is potentially permanent.

## *90. The Case of the Double Bovie*

The patient was a 48-year-old woman whose breast biopsies had shown invasive lobular carcinoma in one breast and lobular carcioma in situ in the other breast. Because of the high risk of bilateral cancer, it was decided to do bilateral mastectomy. In order to conserve operating time, the attending surgeon would do the mastectomy on one side, and the chief resident would do the other side.

Only one electrosurgery unit was available, but it was a new model that had electrical outlets for two separate Bovies with a manual switch on each. Neither the attending surgeon nor the chief resident was aware that activating either switch would activate both electrodes.

During the procedure, the attending surgeon put his Bovie probe down, leaving the tip in contact with the skin of the lower chest. The chief resident, who did not realize that he would be activating both units, activated his own switch in preparation for using his Bovie to dissect the breast from the chest wall. The result was a burn from the second tip. The injury was not major and was easily excised; therefore, no major harm was done.

The source of this error was in the lack of understanding of the new Bovie unit. This would have been readily apparent if either the attending surgeon or the chief resident had read the operating manual.

Not only that, it is not a good practice to allow a Bovie tip to rest in contact with the skin. Most Bovie units come with an insulated plastic sheath, and the Bovie probe should always be placed in that sheath when it is not being used for its intended purpose.

## *91. The Dangers of Subclavian Puncture*

The patient was a 52-year-old man who was scheduled to undergo an urgent operation for an expanding abdominal aortic aneurysm.

Because of anticipated management problems, it was decided to place a subclavian catheter preoperatively, and this was done using a J-wire technique. A moderate amount of difficulty was noted in placing the catheter, but afterward it appeared to be functioning well. The patient, however, soon developed signs of shock, and his "central venous pressures" as measured through the catheter were quite high. A diagnosis of cardiogenic shock was made and the patient was treated with Dopamine to support his cardiac output.

During the course of this management a chest X-ray was taken, which showed an apparent accumulation of fluid in the right chest. This led to some confusion since the subclavian puncture was done on the left side, and the treatment for cardiogenic shock continued.

Shortly thereafter a more experienced physician correctly diagnosed a right hemothorax. This was promptly drained with a chest tube, and the patient's vital signs were restored. The patient subsequently underwent an uneventful resection of his aortic aneurysm.

The errors in this case were both in technique and in management. Obviously, the hemothorax originated from a perforation of the superior vena cava with the J-wire. Any resistance in the placement of a J-wire should be regarded with a great deal of suspicion. Moreover, it must be remembered that complications from subclavian puncture can occur on the opposite side, although they are far more common on the side of the subclavian puncture itself. The other error in management resulted from relying too much on the information obtained by pressure readings from the subclavian catheter. Fortunately, this error was corrected before irreversible damage had occurred.

## 92. *Airway Obstruction in an Intubated Patient*

The patient was a 24-year-old woman who had 30 percent second and third degree burns of the upper part of her body, including the face. In addition, she had severe smoke inhalation, requiring endotracheal intubation immediately on arrival in the emergency room.

During the following two weeks, the patient was supported on a ventilator and was reasonably stable, although her pulmonary function had not improved sufficiently for her to be extubated. Consequently, consideration was given to doing an elective tracheostomy, especially since the nurses reported that they were having some difficulty in suctioning the tube.

The day before the tracheostomy was scheduled, the patient suddenly deteriorated: she became cyanotic and her blood pressure dropped. She was disconnected from the respirator and ventilated by hand, and it was noted that a great deal of pressure was required to expand her lungs, and her breath sounds were difficult to hear.

The possibility of tension pneumothorax was considered, but bilateral needle aspirations revealed no evidence of pneumothorax. An emergency chest X-ray showed the endotracheal tube to be in good position with no kinks in it. The possibililty of a partial obstruction of the tube was considered, but because of the massive swelling around the face there was some concern about changing the tube for fear of being unable to insert a new one. Therefore, a flexible fiberoptic bronchoscope was passed down through the endotracheal tube to inspect its lumen. The endoscopist saw no evidence of obstruction; he passed the bronchoscope easily into the main stem bronchi and saw no evidence of bronchial obstruction either. The cause of the ventilation disturbance was still a mystery.

The patient's $pCO_2$ was rising rapidly and was, at this point, over 100. In desperation and not knowing what else to do, the surgeon decided to change the endotracheal tube in spite of anticipated difficulties. The original tube was found to be about 50 percent occluded with mucous. Upon changing the tube, the patient's blood gases returned to normal.

The lesson to be learned from this case is that, when a patient with an endotracheal tube that has been present for more than a few days develops signs of partial airway obstruction, the tube must be the primary suspect. The possibility of tension pneumothorax was reasonable in view of the physical findings but was easily ruled out with a needle aspiration. The physicians were at least temporarily deceived when they could easily pass a bronchoscope and saw no evidence of obstruction; the optical distortions involved in bronchoscopy made the lumen appear larger than it actually was. The negative impression of the endoscopist confirmed the lack of accuracy of that method for assessing the patency of an endotracheal tube.

The other important consideration they should have thought about is that a partially obstructed airway will typically result in rapid decompensation as soon as the critical level is reached. The patient's blood oxygen levels were maintained by high levels of inspired oxygen, but the poor air flow resulted in rising levels of $CO_2$.

Fortunately, the problem was ultimately recognized and corrected before irreversible damage was done.

## *93. Another Central Catheter Misadventure*

A 47-year-old woman had pancreatitis and a pancreatic abscess that required open drainage. She had been responding to treatment quite well and was recovering in the hospital and receiving intravenous hyperalimentation.

While walking in the hall, she began feeling a little light-headed. The nurse had her sit down in her room and took her blood pressure, which was only 80 systolic. The nurse had her get back in bed and she rechecked: the blood pressure was 70. Within a few minutes it was 50.

The house officer was called. He stopped her hyperalimentation and increased her fluid infusion, without response. The patient was becoming severely short of breath, and an endotracheal tube was inserted. Shortly thereafter the patient had an apparent cardiac arrest, and rescusitative efforts were instituted. The working diagnosis during these maneuvers was a pulmonary embolism, and the patient was given 10,000 units of heparin.

As the situation continued to worsen, the resident decided he should rule out tension pneumothorax and bilateral pneumothorax. He tapped both sides of the chest with a needle; no air returned from either tap, so he decided to tap the pericardium. The pericardial tap returned clear fluid that was slightly bloodstained and had a very high glucose content. Immediately following the pericardial tap the patient's cardiovascular status improved.

In retrospect, it seems obvious that the patient had pericardial tamponade, but the diagnosis was missed until she almost died because no one suspected that it was a possibility. A retrospective review of her chest X-ray plus chemical analysis of the pericardial fluid revealed the etiology. The patient's hyperalimentation catheter had perforated the atrium and the fluid infusion was going into the pericardial space.

The significance of this error in diagnosis is not only that the resident should have been aware of the possibility of an unusual perforation from a central catheter, but that the tip of the catheter should have been in the superior vena cava instead of in the atrium.

## *94. It Is Possible to Be Too Careful*

The patient was a 16-year-old boy who had been in a motor vehicle accident and was admitted by way of the emergency room with a fracture of the mandible and the zygoma. The following day he was taken to the operating room for open reduction and internal fixation of his zygomatic fracture and a closed reduction and interdental fixation of the mandible fracture.

Because of the need for interdental fixation, a nasoendotracheal tube was used. Postoperatively, because the patient had a substantial amount of edema, it was elected to leave the nasotracheal tube in place while he recovered from anesthesia. The procedure took place late in the afternoon, therefore the plan was to wait until the following morning to remove the tube. During the night the patient was very uncomfortable with the tube in place, and because of this he required heavy sedation.

At approximately five o'clock the following morning, the nurse observed that the patient appeared to be having an epileptic seizure. She disconnected the tracheal tube and ventilated the patient using an ambubag. After one or two minutes the patient recovered from his seizure. At that point she noticed that the tubing had become disconnected from the ventilator. The ventilator tubing was reconnected and the equipment was later checked by a technician, who found that the alarm was not working. The patient was extubated later that morning and made an uneventful recovery.

This patient narrowly avoided a catastrophe. If the nurse had not been standing at his bedside when the seizure occurred, he would almost certainly have died. In retrospect, the physician's decision to leave the endotracheal tube in place overnight seems reasonable but probably represents overtreatment. There is a natural reluctance to remove an endotracheal tube from a patient who is unable to breathe through the normal nasal airway if his mouth cannot be opened. Once the patient recovered from anesthesia, he no longer needed the tube and it was producing a great deal of restlessness, which is probably what led to its becoming dislodged from the ventilator.

There is also a natural reluctance to remove tubes late in the day, because if the patient has a problem, it is more likely to develop later in the evening when there aren't as many people around to deal with it. In this case, however, that extra bit of caution almost led to a disaster.

We have a natural tendency to rely on our sophisticated medical equipment with ventilators and alarms, but it is well to remember that these are mechanical devices and are subject to failure. Advanced and sophisticated life support equipment is certainly an advantage of modern medical care, but they should be reserved for those cases in which they are absolutely necessary.